# Social Rules for Kids

*27 Principles for Mastering Respectful Interactions and Developing Self-Esteem, Emotional Intelligence, and Positive Relationships*

# Table of Contents

# Introduction Letter to Parents

Dear Parents,

It's normal to be concerned about your child's social development. Every child is different, and some children find it more challenging than others to learn the rules of social interactions.

Your child might be dealing with issues like bullying or struggling to connect with peers. Some children are also naturally shy, while others don't know how to start a conversation or communicate with others. Understand that this is normal. At this age, your little one is still navigating the world around them and learning how to interact with others. Naturally, they struggle; *no one is born with social skills.* They will learn them along the way. This book is to help children learn social rules and give them practical, fun tips to improve their interactions with others.

You should track your child's progress, but you should not put pressure on them. Pressure can lead to anxiety and develop or worsen social anxiety. You must encourage them but wait until they are ready to share. Remember, while your child needs to interact with others, there is seldom a need to force them to interact with specific individuals. Don't worry about your child; they will learn everything they need to become more social and communicative, and you will notice changes in them that will make you beam with pride.

This book will help your child improve their social skills and emotional intelligence, communicate better, and develop confidence. Thank you for buying it for your child!

# Introduction Letter to Children

Hey Kids,

This book is here to help you. It will help you get along better with everyone at school, help you speak up in class without being afraid, and you skills that even grownups need, too!

You've been given this book because people love you. It's not because there's something wrong with you. We all need a bit of help now and then. Sometimes parents and teachers have many other things to do, so this book lets you work on things in your own time, in your own way.

You will learn many interesting things in this book that will make socializing and having conversations with other people easy and fun. You will not dread talking to others anymore or get nervous when speaking in front of your class. You will be so good at it that you will easily chat with your classmates and make friends. For example, you will discover what empathy is and how to put yourself in other people's shoes. This great ability will make you understand your family and friends better.

Do you know that you can tell what someone wants to say even when they are silent? No, you don't have to be Harry Potter or learn the perfect spell to read people's minds. You can just notice their face and body, and you will understand how they are feeling. You will learn these tricks in this book and more! The fun doesn't end here; you will also learn cool ways to control your emotions and reactions, make friends, solve problems, be more confident, and (this might be the best part) you will learn how to stand up to bullies and protect yourself from them. Awesome, right?

Never be afraid to ask questions and seek help from a trusted adult; they want to help you. Share your progress with your parents and show off what you can do.

The tips in this book are easy and fun and include activities you can do with your friends.

# Section 1: Social Interactions

We all have to interact socially, even when we don't always want to. These interactions can be like minefields.

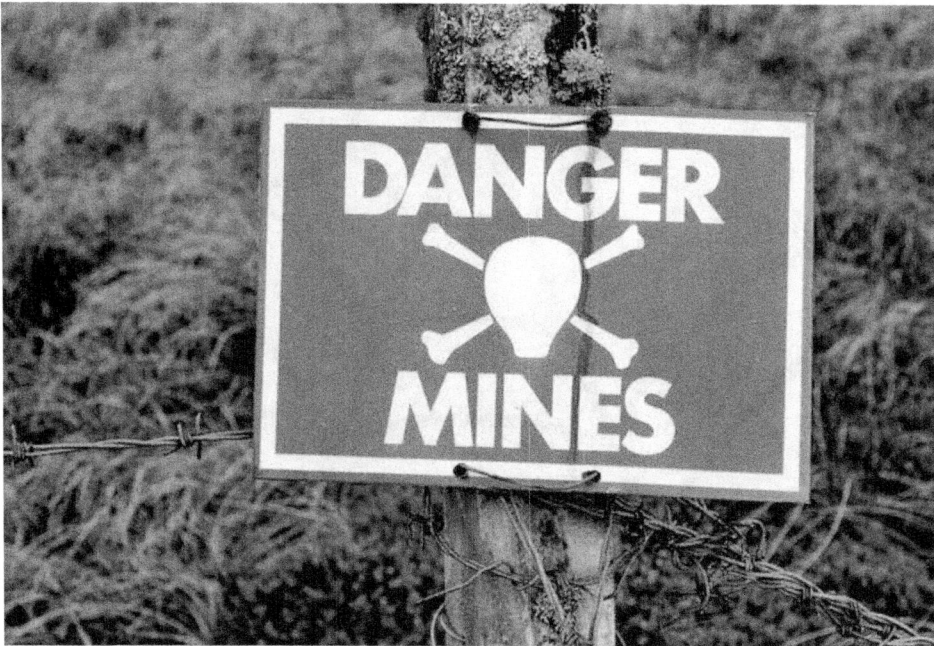

Interactions can sometimes feel like minefields.
*https://pixabay.com/photos/sign-danger-beware-mines-dangerous-5458066/*

Remember, everyone messes up sometimes. Think of times when your friends have said and done things that upset you without intention. There's no easy way to handle every interaction.

However, three principles can help you: respect, politeness, and kindness. Being kind first makes a significant difference. These three and all the other principles (in each section) are like a web of social skills; they're stronger together.

EMOTIONAL AWARENESS

NON-JUDGMENT

CONFLICT RESOLUTION

CLEAR COMMUNICATION

POLITENESS

KINDNESS

RESPECT

SELF-REFLECTION

COOPERATION

LOYALTY

REFUSE

RESPECT FOR OTHERS' BELIEFS

ACTIVE LISTENING

ACCEPTING DIFFERENCES

EMOTIONAL REGULATION

NEGOTIATION

SHARING

EMPATHY

COMPROMISE

NON-VERBAL CUES

CULTURAL SENSITIVITY

POSITIVE SELF-TALK

UNDERSTANDING

REPORT

RECOGNIZE

GOAL-SETTING

ASSERTIVENESS

27 PRINCIPLES

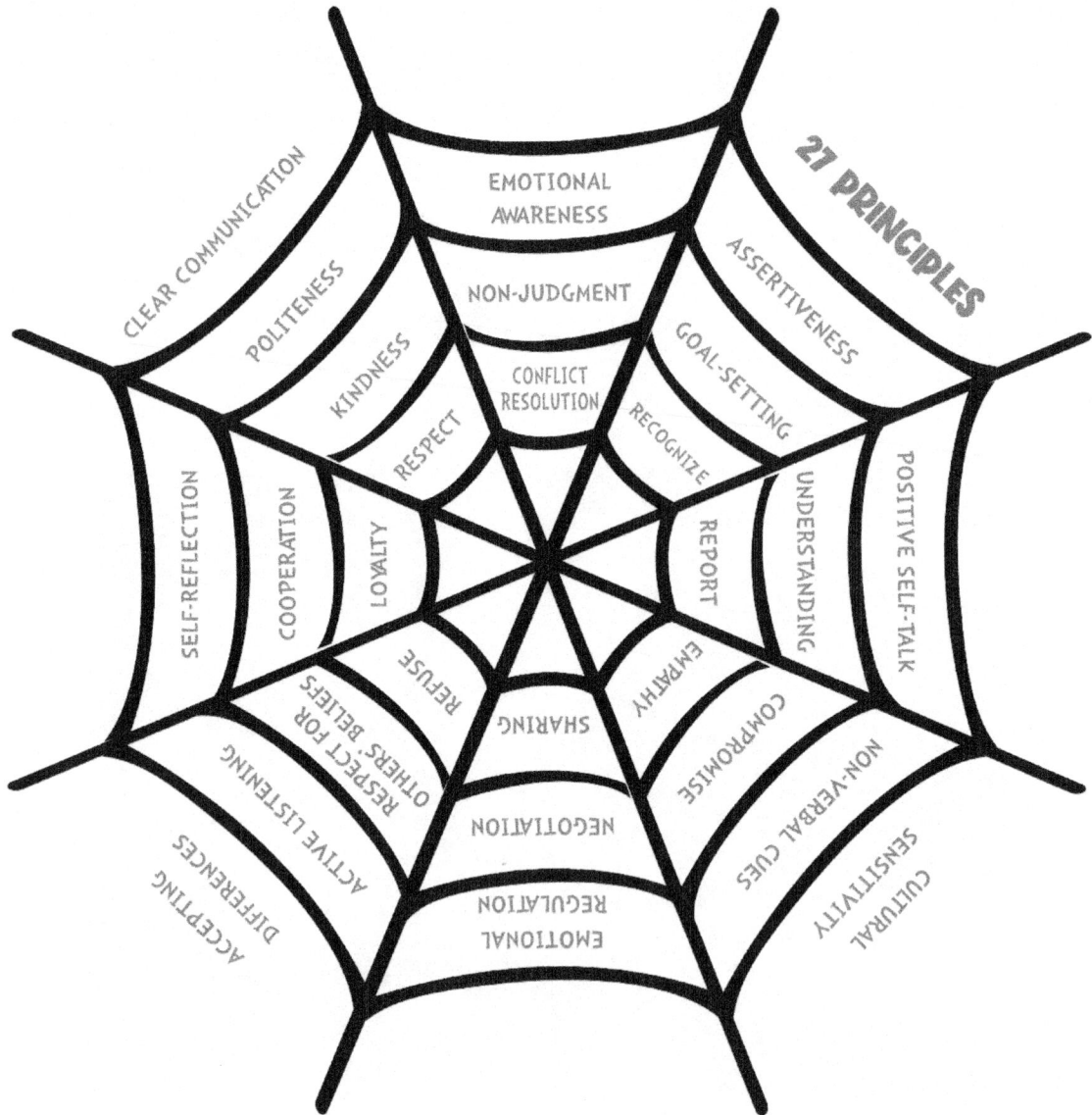

## Principle 1: Respect

In this case, respect doesn't mean placing somebody above you. You might be asked to be respectful by teachers, meaning to do what you're told. However, this isn't that type of respect. The other definition is to care about other people's feelings, wishes, rights, and traditions – this is the right one.

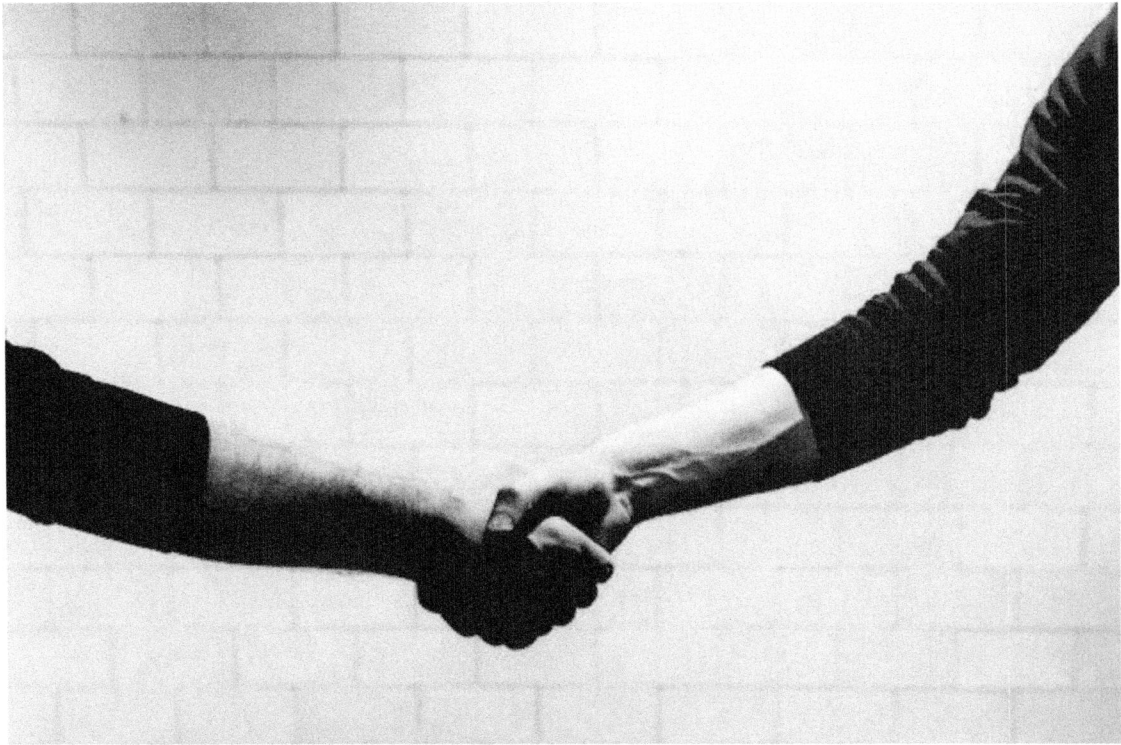

Everyone should be treated with respect.

This respect can and should be mutual. You should treat everyone with respect. Watch how adults treat servers in a restaurant; you will notice that some are respectful and others aren't.

Here are four exercises to help you be more respectful of others:

1. **Role-Playing.** Role-playing is fun and helps you be more creative. Create a situation where respect is needed, and act it out with your friends. One person can pretend to be new in a class, pick a topic you disagree on, like a cartoon plotline, and practice discussing it respectfully.

2. **Respect Circle.** Stand together in a circle with your friends. Everyone says something respectful about the person on their left, such as "I love hearing about your family's traditions."

3. **Respect Statements.** Write down respectful things you want to work on, starting with, "I will." You could ask your parents for ideas.

4. **Respect Words.** Write down as many words associated with respect as possible. This exercise helps you define respect better so you can do it better.

# Principle 2: Politeness

Being polite is about following rules. Somebody has probably told you to mind your manners, which means saying "please" and "thank you." These little words might not seem like much, but they're the ball bearings in a bike wheel. They keep everything moving smoothly.

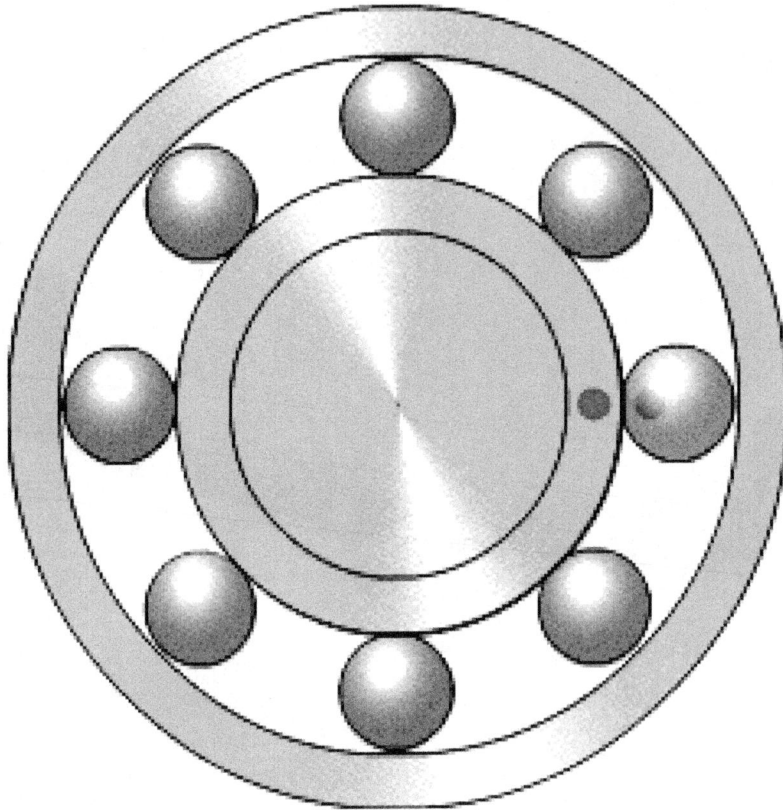

Being polite keeps everything moving smoothly, like ball bearings.
*PlusMinus, CC BY-SA 3.0 <http://creativecommons.org/licenses/by-sa/3.0/>, via Wikimedia Commons:*
*https://commons.wikimedia.org/wiki/File:BallBearing.gif*

You can practice being polite with your friends and your family. It's easy not to be polite when you know somebody, but you can get out of the habit.

Here are four exercises to practice politeness:

1. **The Rude Noise.** Get together with your friends, and make a rude noise when you catch a friend not being polite. Think of imitating the "wrong buzzer" from your favorite game show.

2. **Good Manners Box.** Have a box and put a piece of paper in it every time you do something polite, like saying please, holding the door for somebody whose hands are full, etc. Ask your parents for a small reward when the box is full.

3. **Write a Thank You Note** to somebody who has done something nice for you (or write one to your parents). Thank you notes are appreciated by grownups, too.

4. **Research Good Manners in Another Culture.** Not everyone does things the same. Get an adult to help you research. (This also helps with respect.)

# Principle 3: Kindness

Kindness is defined in the dictionary as being "friendly, generous, and considerate."

Being kind is showing you care for people. Your family and friends don't know you care about them unless you tell them and show them. They can't read your mind.

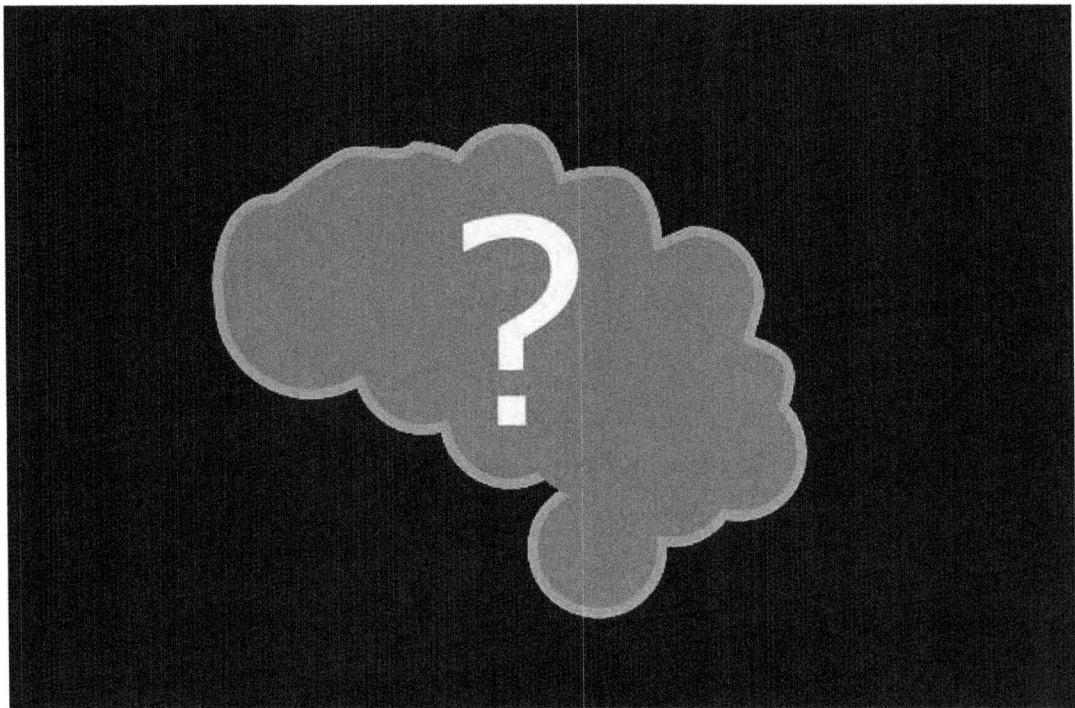

You must think carefully about what you want to say and ensure it sounds kind.
https://pixabay.com/illustrations/brain-question-thinking-4721936/

In social interactions, you must think about everything you say and ensure it shows you care. Mean is the opposite of kind. Consider the mean things you've heard and said this week.

Here are four exercises to practice kindness:

1. **Do a Random Act of Kindness.** Do something for somebody you don't know very well. It might be picking up something a stranger dropped and making sure they get it back or letting somebody go ahead of you through a doorway.

2. **Compliment Circle.** This is like the respect circle, except you compliment the person on your left instead, like "You did well in math class" or "I love how you did your hair today."

3. **Compliment Yourself.** You have to be kind to yourself to be kind to others. Say something to yourself you would say to a good friend every day.

4. **Practice T.H.I.N.K.** Before you open your mouth, ask if what you're about to say is True, Helpful, Inspiring, Necessary, and Kind. Sometimes, you must say something harsh because it's necessary, but it must also be helpful and worded in kindness.

# Section 2: Empathy and Understanding

*Disclaimer for the parents: This section discusses concepts like judgment and bias. If you are worried that the content of this chapter may affect your child's beliefs, ask them to skip it.*

It can be challenging to have empathy and understanding – thinking about how others view a situation. But think about the last book you read. When you read a book, you see the situation through someone else's eyes, who might be quite different from you. That's *empathy.*

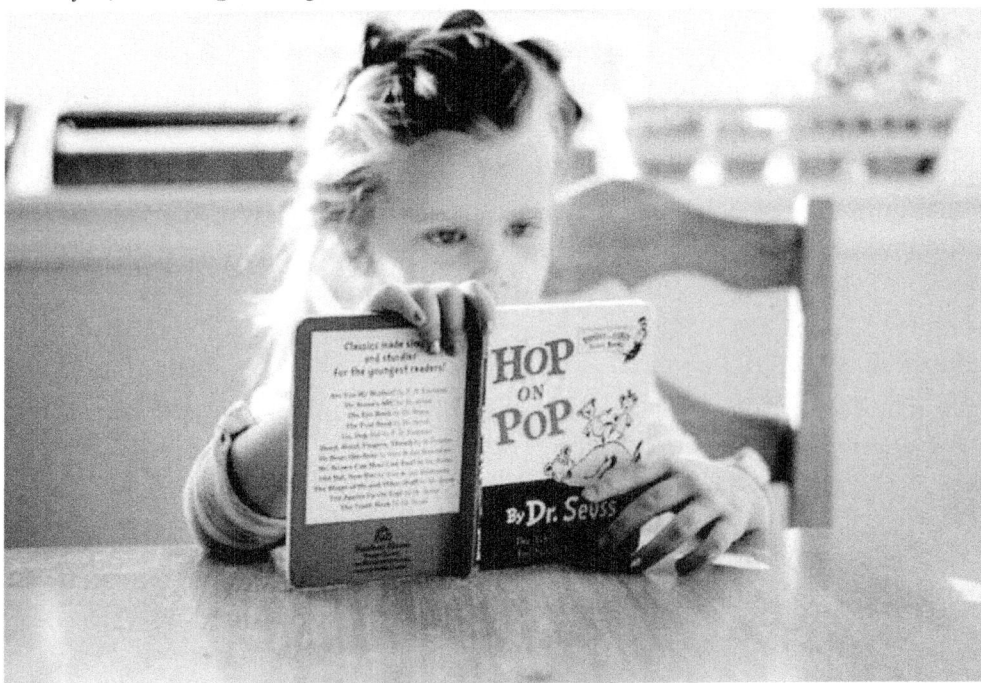

When you read a book, you see situations from a different perspective.

The three principles are empathy, understanding, and non-judgment. It's easy to play judge and jury on what others do, especially if it hurts you. Not everyone who hurts you does it *on purpose.*

Showing empathy, understanding, and non-judgment helps you interact with others, so it gets them on your side and avoids fights.

# Principle 4: Empathy

It's not a science fiction book you read or show you watched where a character can sense other people's feelings. Empathy is imagining what someone else feels. Some people find this easier than others, and that's okay. Have you heard the expression "Put yourself in someone else's shoes"? Well, this is empathy. It is the ability to know how someone else feels, even if you have never been in their situation.

It means when somebody else is suffering, you can imagine what it's like to be them, helping you treat them in a way that you help without hurting them more. For example, your friend is sad because their grandfather is sick. Even if both of your grandparents are healthy and none of your family members was ever sick before, you will still understand the pain and sadness your friend is going through. So you will be there for them, support them, and listen when they want to talk.

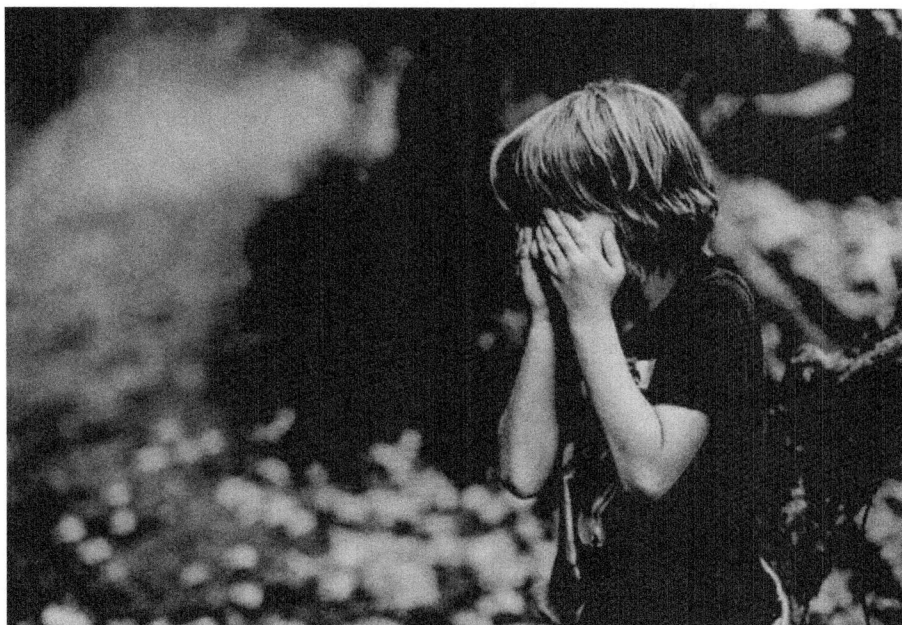

An example of empathy is that when someone is crying, you can imagine how they feel.
*https://unsplash.com/photos/svSclyGGJv4?utm_source=unsplash&utm_medium=referral&utm_content=creditShareLink*

Some people struggle with empathy and might need a lot of help with it, perhaps from a professional.

Here are four exercises to improve empathy:

1. **Read a Book about Someone Very Different from You.** Ask your parents or the school librarian to help you pick a suitable book. Even better, get your friends to read the same book so you can discuss the character and story.

2. **Play Emotional Charades with Your Friends.** Emotional charades is a game where one person acts out an emotion, and the others must guess what it is. Then trade-off.

3. **Make an Empathy Map.** Choose an emotion, then write down everything you might hear, think and feel, say and do, and see if you felt that way.

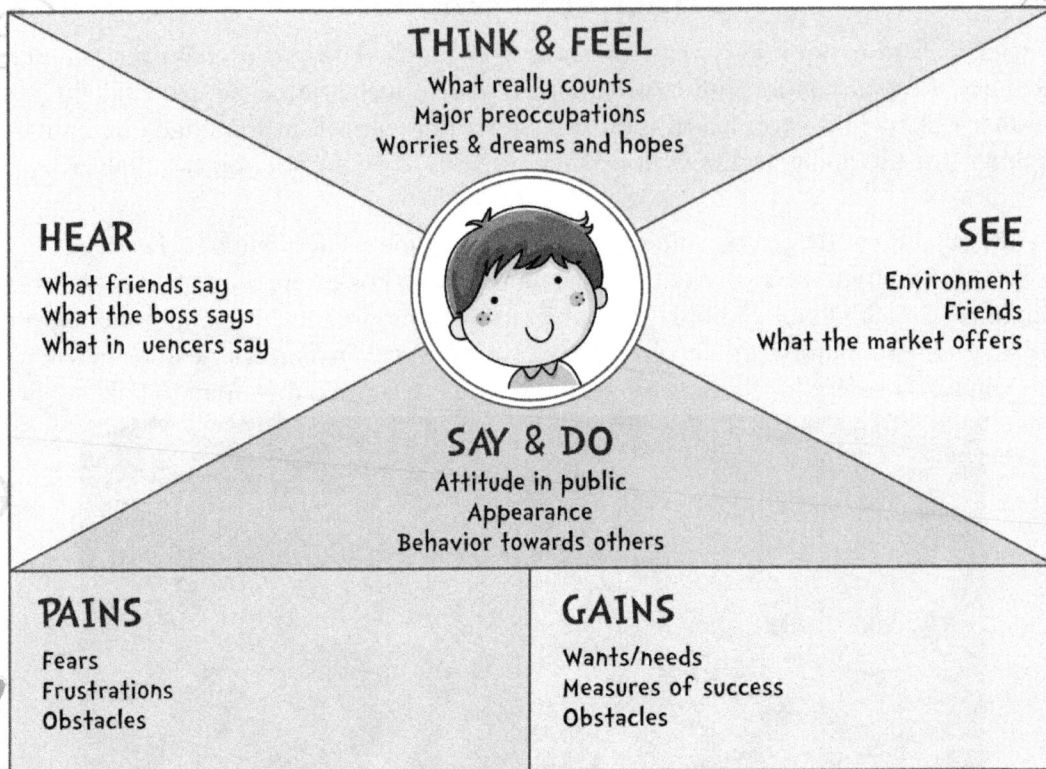

```
                    THINK & FEEL
                    What really counts
                    Major preoccupations
                    Worries & dreams and hopes


  HEAR                                              SEE
  What friends say                         Environment
  What the boss says                          Friends
  What in uencers say              What the market offers


                    SAY & DO
                    Attitude in public
                    Appearance
                    Behavior towards others


  PAINS                            GAINS

  Fears                            Wants/needs
  Frustrations                     Measures of success
  Obstacles                        Obstacles
```

4. **Take Responsibility for Something.** Talk to your parents about a pet or a plant in your room. Or, practice "taking care" of a stuffed animal or get a phone app with a virtual pet.

# Principle 5: Understanding

In this case, "understanding" means being aware and tolerant of other people's feelings. It's a step beyond empathy because empathy is knowing what they feel; understanding is allowing them to feel it.

For example, Philip is really mad his favorite show got canceled. You think that show is stupid. Empathy is knowing they're mad. Understanding is accepting they're mad even though you don't agree.

Things that upset you might not upset others.

How to improve understanding:

1. **Story Mistakes.** Ask a friend or trusted adult to read you a familiar story and to make mistakes. Tell them how many you spotted. It helps you listen to what people say better.

2. **Make a Values List.** Write down those values that are important to you. Remember, everyone else has one too. This list helps you understand yourself better.

3. **Have a Debate.** Pick a topic you won't get too heated about, and debate with a friend. Switch sides. Debating something you don't agree with helps you understand other people's perspectives.

4. **Make a Friend Strengths List.** Pick one of your friends and write a list of their strengths and good qualities. Consider asking them to do the same for you.

# Principle 6: Non-Judgment

Non-judgment can be the hardest to practice. Judging people is natural- even judging *yourself.*

The world can seem very judgmental at times. You get graded – a judgment on how well you're doing.

However, this is not what non-judgment means. It means not judging others by your *biases.* Everyone has biases (in favor of or against something); you pick them up from your parents and the adults around you, whether they want to teach them.

Practicing non-judgment starts with knowing how you judge people.

Here are some exercises to help you be less judgmental:

1. **Bias Exercise.** Get a picture of a person. Write down the things you think about them right away. Repeat with several pictures. Then, find the people with whom you have common negative reactions.

2. **Keep a Judgment Diary.** Whenever you have a thought like "She is too fat," write it down. This diary helps you catch these thoughts before they get out where others can hear them. Rewrite them as something positive, such as "She is very confident in her body."

3. **Read a Book You Think Won't Be Fun Based on the Cover.** Write down everything you liked about it. Sometimes you will be right about the book, but often you won't. It helps you judge less with first impressions.

4. **Play the "Wrong" Game.** Write down whenever you think, "That's wrong" about something somebody did. Then, write down a reason that person might have done it. If in doubt, ask your parents.

# Section 3: Effective Communication

Do you always understand what your friends say? Do they sometimes think you said something completely different? Everyone messes up communication sometimes, even people who are good at it.

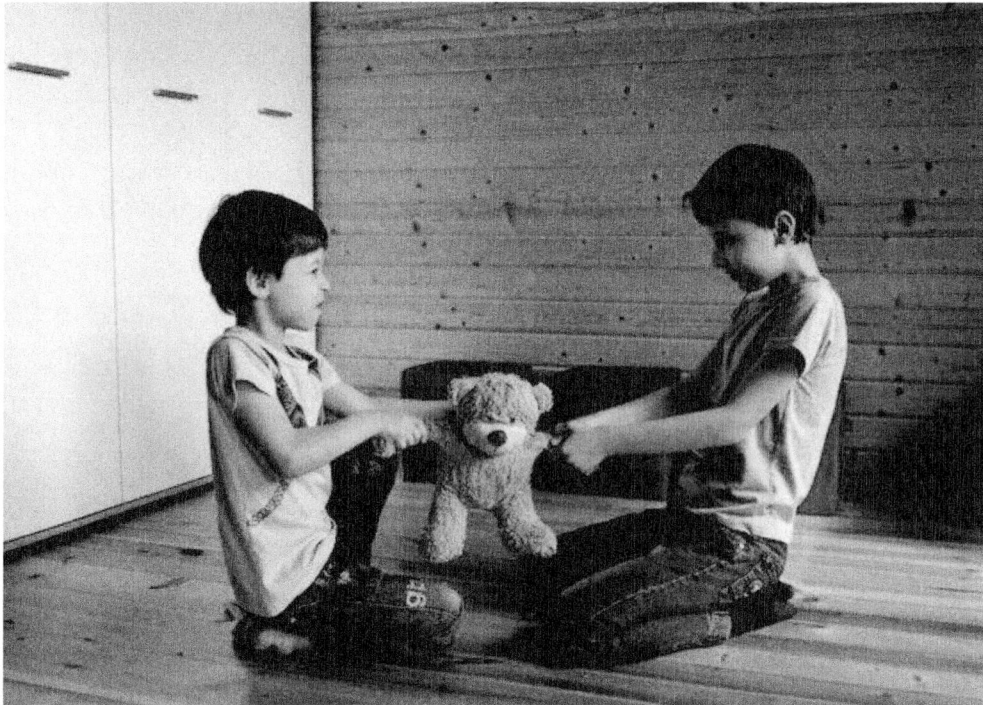

Learning to communicate effectively can help you avoid disagreements.
https://www.pexels.com/photo/angry-little-brothers-fighting-and-pulling-toy-to-sides-4140308/

You can learn to say what you mean better and understand what others say. Your brain has communication filters, which include emotions and biases.

Three things are needed for good communication: clear talking, nonverbal (not spoken) cues, and active listening. Most of these exercises need other people, so rope in friends, siblings, family, etc., and let's get some practice.

# Principle 7: Clear Communication

You can't always control how people hear you, but practicing clear communication helps ensure it isn't your fault when they misunderstand.

Fun communication exercises:

1. **Describe and Show.** Pick a topic. Grab an item related to that topic, like a toy or a garden trowel, and describe it in a few sentences to your friends.

2. **Back to Back.** You can play this with a friend. Get an item, but don't let your friend see it. Sit back to back and describe the object. They have to guess what it is. Then switch.

3. **Communication Filters Game.** On the worksheet, write down everything you can think of that makes communicating hard, like being angry, not liking the person, etc. Write something you can do about it in the right column, like waiting to talk until you've calmed down.

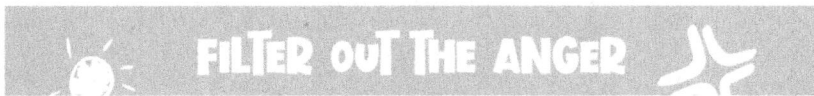

## FILTER OUT THE ANGER

The upset brain thinks

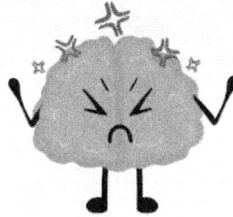

| Okay to say | Filter it out |
| --- | --- |
| | |
| | |
| | |
| | |
| | |
| | |
| | |
| | |
| | |
| | |

4. **Play Telephone**. It's a classic game played with a group of friends. Stand or sit in a line. The person at one end of the line makes up a sentence and whispers it to the next person, who whispers it to the next, and so on, until the last person in the line. The last person at the other end says the sentence out loud. It's often very funny, but it also shows how easily miscommunications happen.

# Principle 8: Non-Verbal Cues

Nonverbal cues are important. For example, if somebody says they're fine, but their shoulders are slumped, and their eyes look sad, they probably aren't fine. You might or might not want to find out why, but you can at least tell they're not fine.

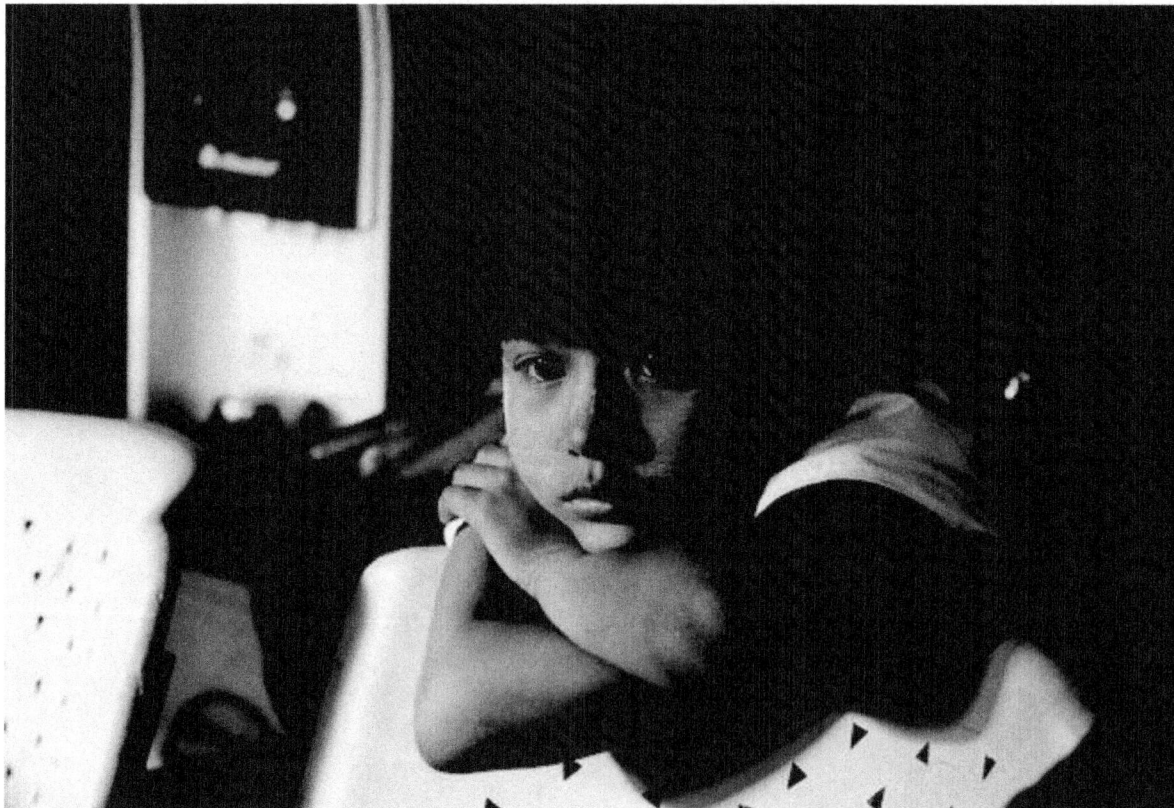

Reading people's body language can be difficult.
*https://unsplash.com/photos/TV1QYUtTxJ8?utm_source=unsplash&utm_medium=referral&utm_content=creditShareLink*

Learning to read other people's body language can be tough, and it's harder for some children than others. If you have a hard time with it, talk to your parents because you might need extra help.

Exercises for nonverbal cues and communication:

1. **Charades**. Playing charades helps you understand and read nonverbal cues. Play with your friends or your parents and siblings.

2. **Play Mime**. Create a role-playing scenario, such as buying something in the store, meeting a new person, etc. The trick is that you must role-play it without saying anything.

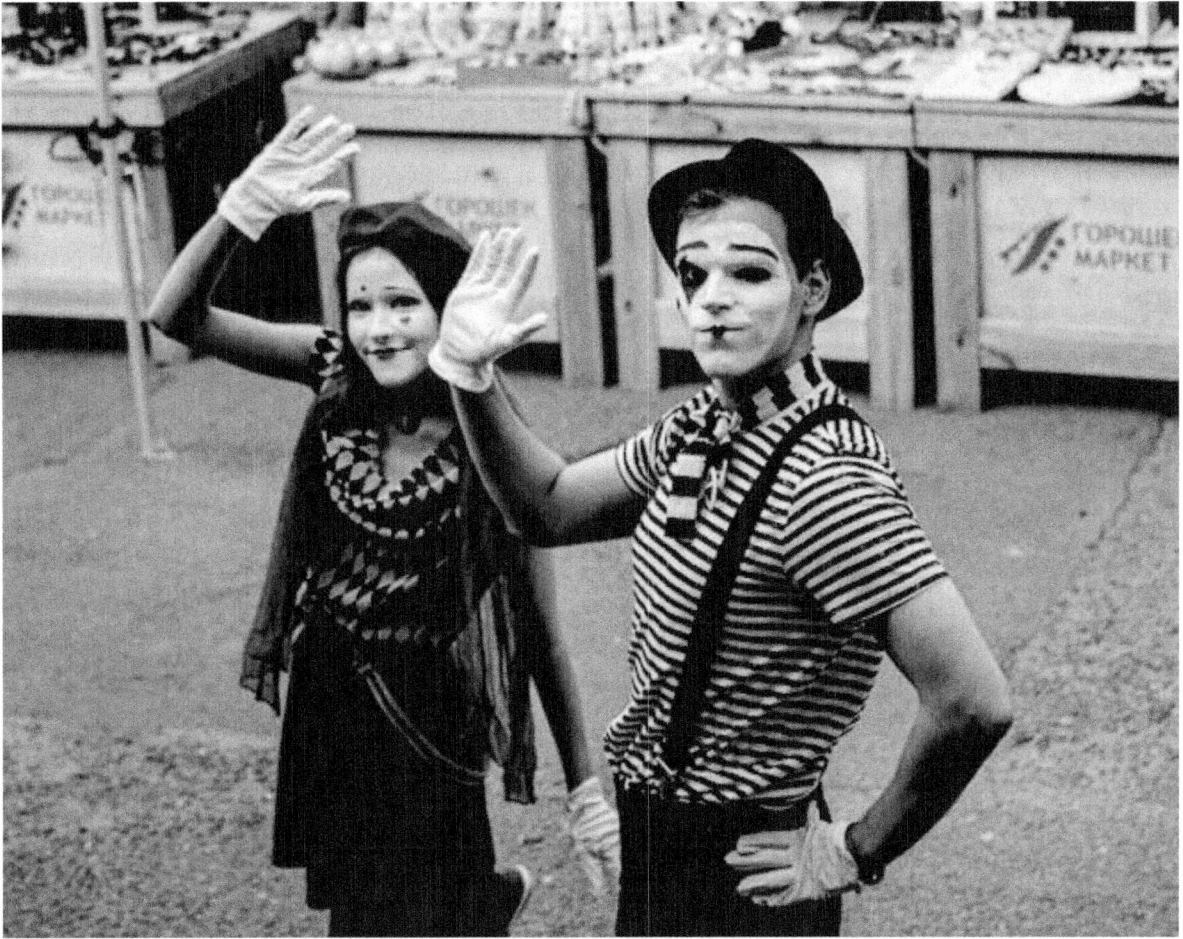

Role-play a scenario without saying anything; that's called mime.

3. **Character Observation.** Play a scene from a TV show without the sound. Work out what the characters are saying to each other, then play it with the sound and see how close you are.

4. **Mirror Game.** Stand facing your friend. One of you does an action, and the other has to copy them. Then switch. This exercise helps you focus on observing people.

# Principle 9: Active Listening

Active listening sounds weird, but it's about paying attention to the person you're talking to and listening and focusing on what they say.

If your attention drifts while listening, you will miss things. Everyone does it, but it can result in bad miscommunication. Missing something can start a fight, so put your phone down during an important conversation.

Here are some exercises to improve active listening:

1. **Simon Says.** The playground game is an excellent way to ensure you listen so you don't end up being "out" quickly. For an extra twist, change "Simon" to another name.

2. **Sound Hunt.** This exercise helps you appreciate the sounds in the world. Using a recording app on your phone, see how many sounds you can find in your backyard or a local park. It helps you notice small sounds and concentrate on focusing, enabling you to listen to others better.

3. **Listen to an Audiobook.** Your library will have audiobooks. It's best to pick a book you haven't read so you don't know what happens. Ask your parents or librarian for ideas.

4. **Round-Robin Story.** Sit in a circle with your friends. Pick somebody to start a story. They tell one sentence, then pass around the circle, with each person adding a sentence. If you don't listen well, the story won't make sense.

# Section 4: Emotional Intelligence

Emotions are tricky things. You must first know your emotions before those of other people. Being aware of your emotions means you can control your responses.

Not your emotions, your responses. Your feelings are perfectly valid. It's okay to be upset that Jerry didn't sit with you at lunch, but it's not okay to go to Jerry and yell at him or tell him you don't like him anymore.

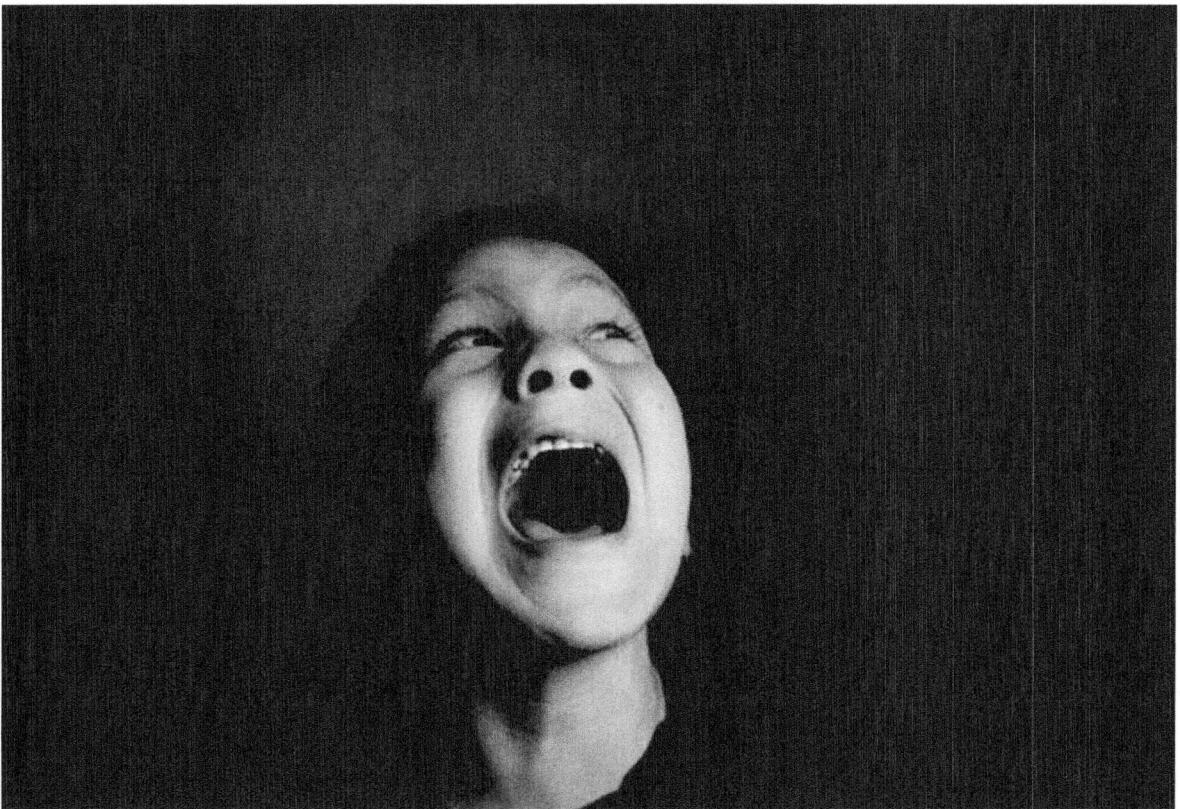

It is important to control your emotions no matter who you're dealing with.

It's essential to wait until you calm down, which can be hard.

So, what is emotional intelligence? It's the skill of understanding your emotions, controlling your emotions, and developing empathy. It's not something you merely have. You must learn it. When you do, you'll do it better your entire life.

People with good emotional intelligence are happier. Think about somebody angry all the time. Are they happy? The chances are no, although they might think making others miserable makes them happy.

There are a few basic things to remember about being smart with emotions, and these include emotional awareness, emotional regulation, and self-reflection. Empathy plays a big role in all this, as well as managing your relationships and staying motivated in the face of problems.

## 5 COMPONENTS OF EMOTIONAL INTELLIGENCE

**1. Self-Awareness**
Be aware of your emotions as they arise.

**2. Self-Regulation**
Manage your impulses, soothe yourself and respond appropriately.

**5. Relationship Management**
Manage others' emotions, organize groups and negotiate solutions.

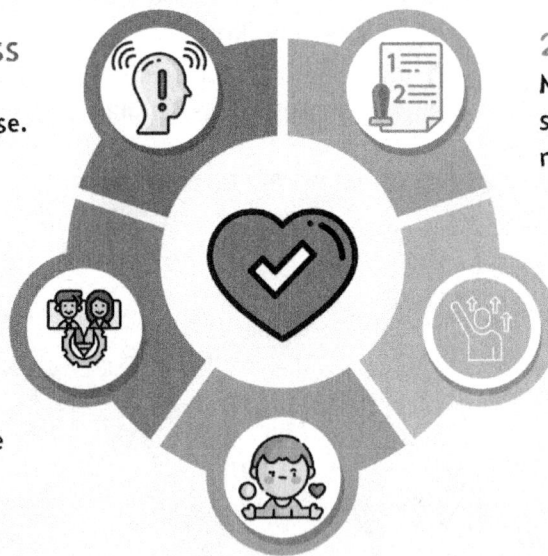

**3. Self-Motivation**
Delay gratification, stay motivated and persistent in face of setbacks.

**4. Empathy**
Understand others' feelings, needs, wants and concerns.

## Principle 10: Emotional Awareness

Knowing your feelings might seem a no-brainer, but think of when you were much younger. Did you always know what an emotion was or what caused it? It's something you have to learn.

Here are some exercises to improve your emotional awareness:

1. **Emotion Identification Quiz.** Look at the nine faces and the nine emotion words. Can you match one to the other? Ask your parents how well you did.

# GUESS THE EMOTION

Instructions: Match the emotion to the correct face.

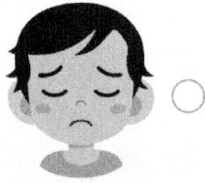 ○ ○ Angry

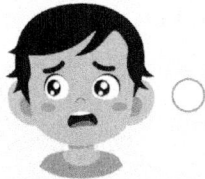 ○ ○ Confused

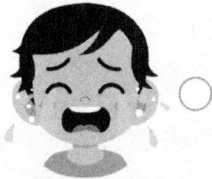 ○ ○ Guilty

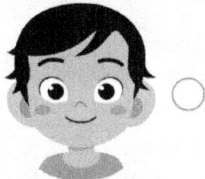 ○ ○ Hurt

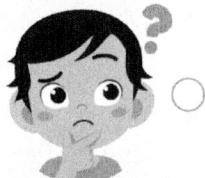 ○ ○ Sad

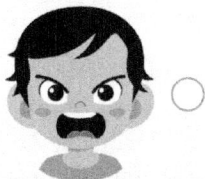 ○ ○ Happy

2. **Take an Emotion and Use It as a Writing Prompt.** Write what a fictional character is likely to do when experiencing that emotion.

3. **Take an Emotion and Draw a Face Matching That Emotion.** You can be silly, for example, by making the face like a dog for more fun.

4. **Play Emotions Pictionary.** One person draws an emotion. The rest must guess what emotion they are drawing.

# Principle 11: Emotional Regulation

Little children show and act on what they feel. If you've been around babies, you know they cry for what they need, and you have to guess what they want.

Hopefully, most grownups around you don't do this because they learned emotional regulation. People who haven't can be unpleasant to deal with.

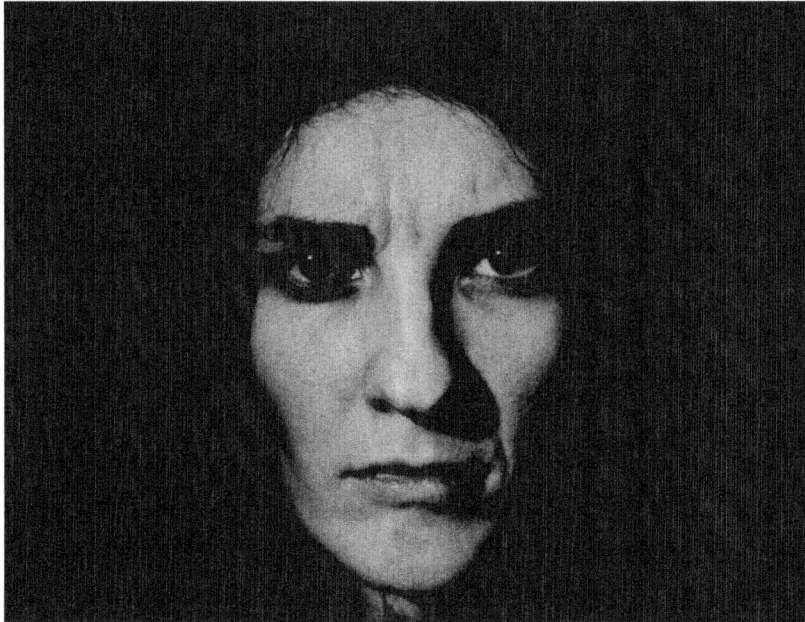

Dealing with grownups who haven't learned emotional regulation can be difficult.
*https://unsplash.com/photos/GT2iUnTfrd8?utm_source=unsplash&utm_medium=referral&utm_content=creditShareLink*

Not being that person means you must learn to identify your emotions and step back from acting on them if necessary. Sometimes, it's fine to be angry about something, but emotional regulation lets you be smart about dealing with that anger.

Some exercises to help improve emotional regulation:

1. **Take a Deep Breath**. Or a few. Paced breathing (inhale for four, exhale for six, or similar) can help. This action turns off the physical reaction of your emotions. Practice this exercise, and use it when you realize you're getting angry or upset.

2. **Use a Stress Relief Ball**. Adults also use these. You can make one with a balloon and some flour. Or have your parents get you one that you like. You can get a stress animal, brain, or computer (great if your computer or phone is the issue). Squeeze the ball when you start getting mad. Clenching and relaxing muscles also tone down emotional reactions.

3. **Play Board Games with Your Friends**. These games help you be a better winner and a better loser. Nobody likes a bad loser. It also helps you practice patience (waiting for a slow person to take their turn) and improve your communication skills.

4. **Learn H.A.L.T**. When you get really mad, ask yourself these four questions: Am I hungry? Am I angry? Am I lonely? Am I tired? If you're hungry, eat something. When you're hungry, your brain sometimes stops properly regulating itself because it lacks energy – and then you get angry. If somebody says they're "hangry," that's what they mean.

# Principle 12: Self-Reflection

Knowing what emotions you feel is the first step. Self-reflection is about knowing when and why you feel particular emotions. Everyone has "hot buttons" that make us angry. Or perhaps you would feel sad if you didn't go outside that day.

Also, It's good to understand the things and people that make you happy. You should always make space for those things in life.

Exercises for self-reflection:

1. **Keep an Emotions Journal.** At the end of the day, write down all your emotions and why you felt them. This exercise helps you identify and deal with things that change your mood, including seeking things and people that make you happy.

2. **Create a "Me" Tree.** Draw a tree on a piece of paper, with space for many leaves. Draw large leaves. Also, draw soil at the bottom. Now do these prompts: Soil: I am supported by... Trunk: I am grateful for... Leaves: I love... This tree helps you know what makes you, you.

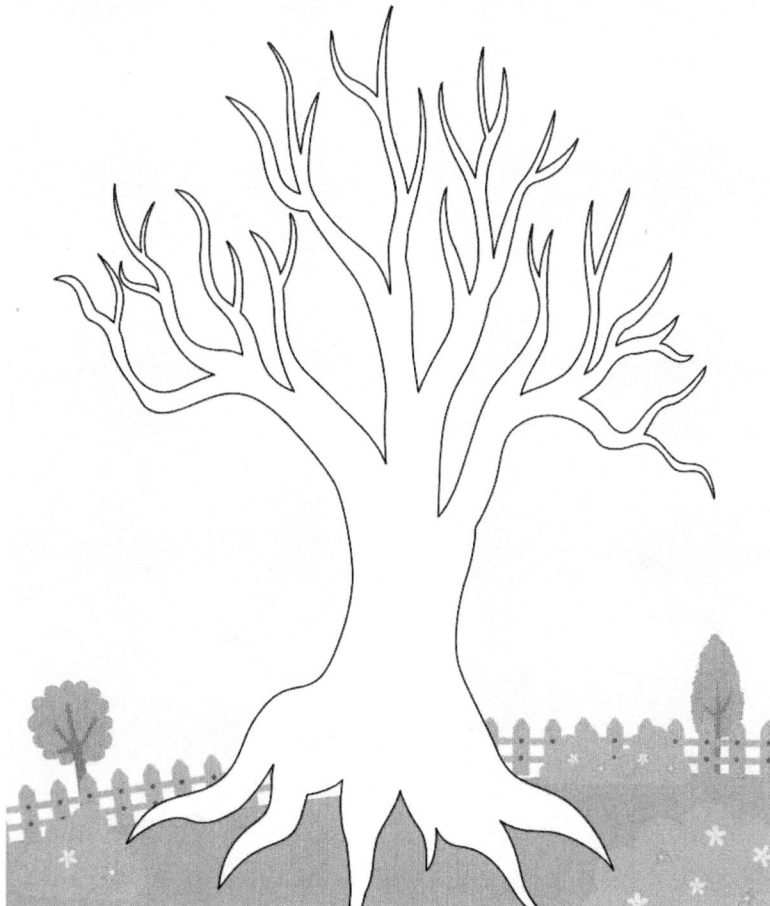

ME TREE

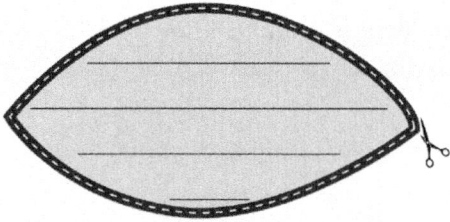
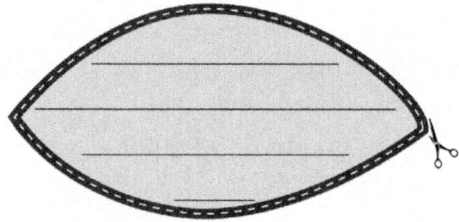
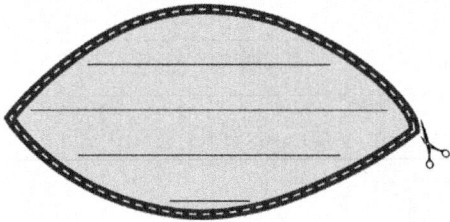
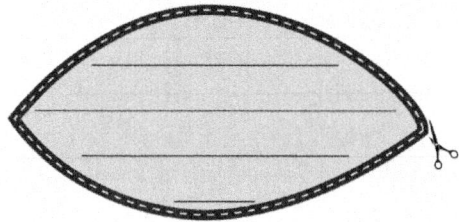
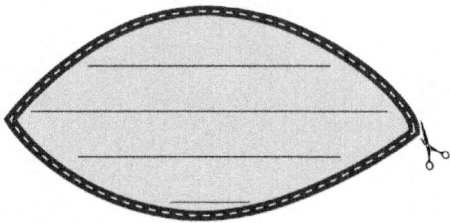
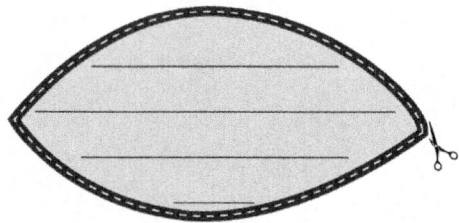
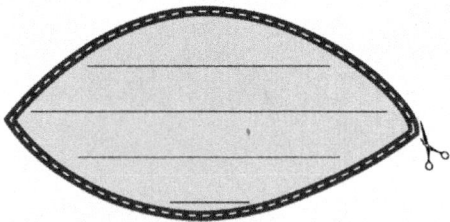
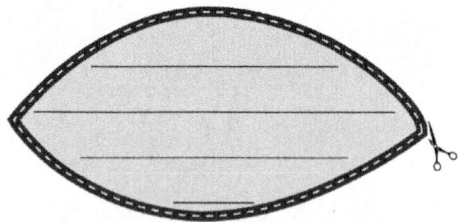
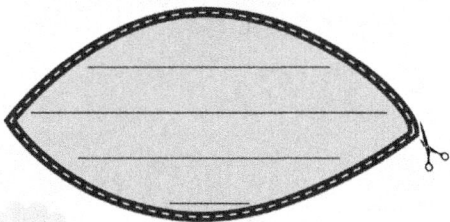
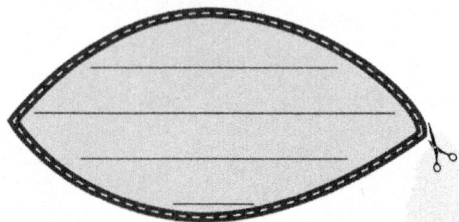
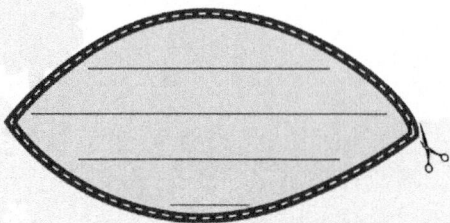
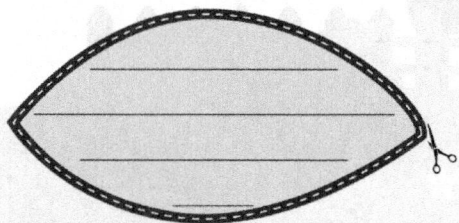

3. **Bag of Beads.** Fill a bag with colorful beads. Each color represents a different emotion. Pull a bead from the bag and either write about things making you feel that emotion or share them with friends.

4. **Make a Gratitude List.** Write down all the things you are grateful for. Keep adding to it. For example, if you make a new friend, add them to the list. Always look for things to be grateful for. You can look at the list when you feel down; it will cheer you up.

So, now that you've finished the chapter, what was your favorite exercise?

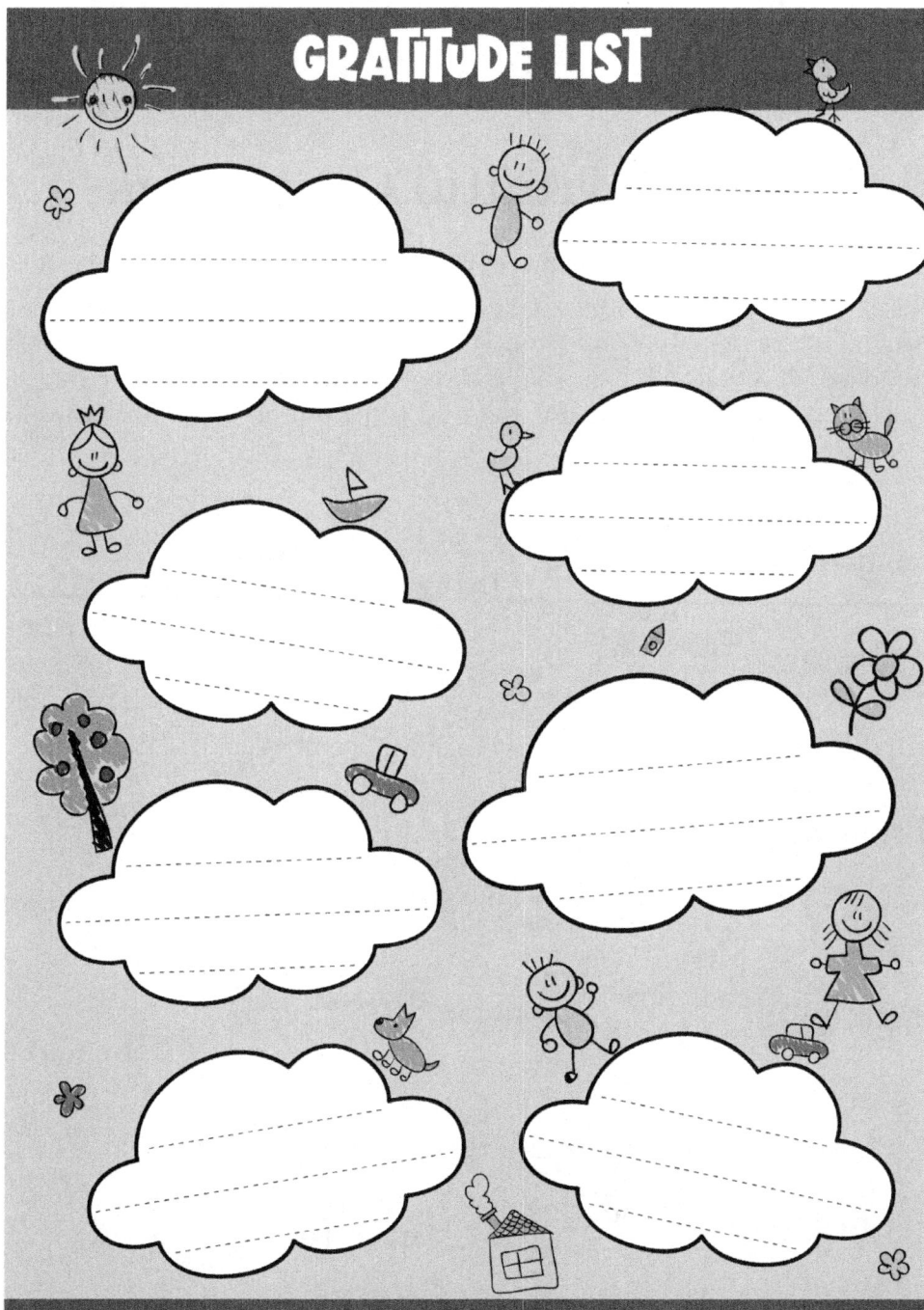

# GRATITUDE LIST

# Section 5: Fruitful Connections

How important are your friends? We all need friends, and while many people don't keep their childhood friends because of various factors, others form lifelong connections.

You need a good relationship with your family, classmates (even those you don't like), and teachers. You don't have to like or get on with everyone, and you certainly don't have to be friends with people you don't like. However, having good friends you trust helps you be happy, do better in school, and always have somebody to talk to.

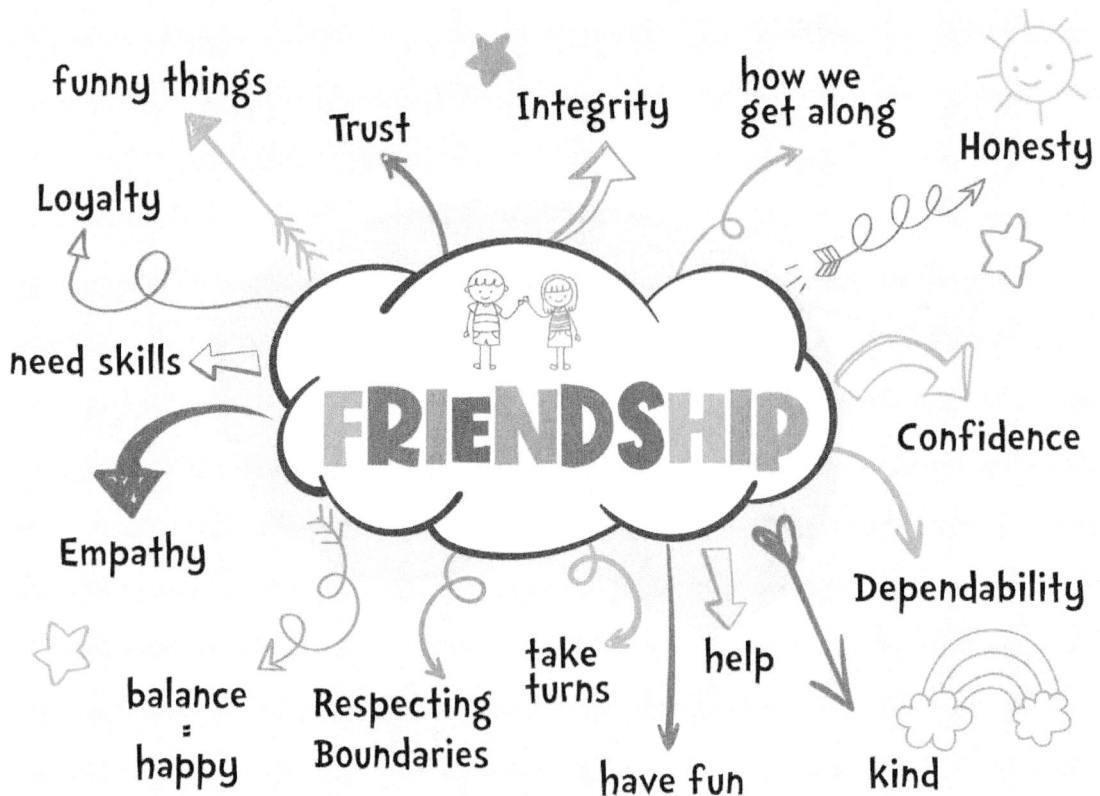

funny things

Trust

Integrity

how we get along

Honesty

Loyalty

need skills

FRIENDSHIP

Confidence

Empathy

Dependability

balance = happy

Respecting Boundaries

take turns

help

have fun

kind

You'll have different friend types in your life, ranging from close confidants to people you share hobbies and activities with, like the other sports team members.

Learn to be a good friend. Go through the above qualities and write down ways you meet them or fall short.

Three important social rules to help you be a good friend are cooperation, sharing, and loyalty.

# Principle 13: Cooperation

Have you been the child who does everything on the group project? It means the rest of the group is failing at cooperation.

Cooperation means doing things together, ensuring nobody carries too much of the load. Teamwork gets things done faster and also helps build sound connections.

Here are some ways to improve cooperation. You'll need your friends for these:

1. **Play a Cooperative Board Game.** While many games have a winner and loser, some games have all the players work together against the game itself, which typically involves several random factors. Cooperative board games often have fun stories for great entertainment.

2. **Blanket Switch.** Get an old blanket and a couple of friends. Put the blanket down and stand on it. You must turn the blanket over without putting a foot off the blanket. It's harder than it sounds.

3. **Cooperative Counting.** You need a big group for this. The aim is to count to 20 by having each child count off the number without an assigned order. If two people say the same number, you have to start over. You can also challenge yourself to see how far you can go.

4. **Word Circle.** Pick one person to start with. They must say a word, and the next person must say a word using the last letter of the previous word. For example, if person one says horse, person two might say egg. You can also determine a theme, *like animals*, so person one says horse, and person two can say elephant. Or have the first word determine the theme (like fruit: apple, elderberry).

# Principle 14: Sharing

Probably, you've been told to share for all your life because *it matters*, but it does not mean you should let down your boundaries. If somebody has a habit of not returning loaned books, you don't have to loan them another book. You aren't in playschool anymore and don't have to share the toys with everyone. However, sharing with people you care about is important.

Sharing doesn't always mean *things*. You should also share your time and interests with your friends.

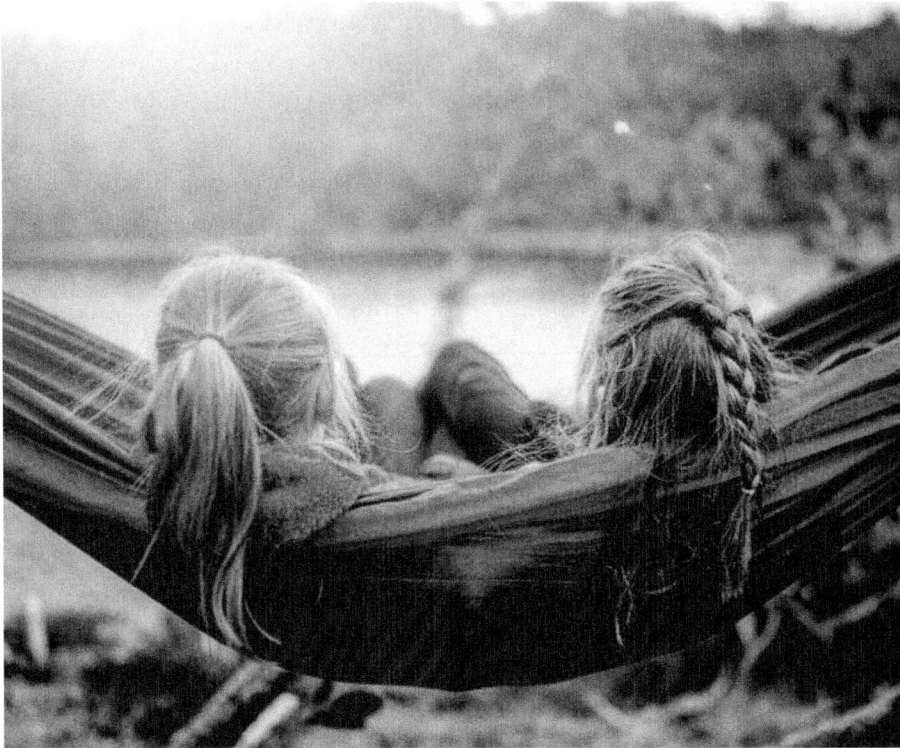

Sharing can just be spending time with your friends.

Here are some exercises to help you share more without losing respect for your boundaries and other people's:

1. **Do a Craft Project with a Friend.** You could draw a picture together. Or the person good at drawing draws and the person good at cutting cuts. It helps you recognize your and other people's strengths.

2. **Arrange a Potluck with Your Friends.** You'll need adult help for this exercise. Everyone makes a dish and brings it to the party – bonus points for making a family recipe or something from your culture.

3. **Trade or Lend Books.** Swapping books with a friend helps you practice sharing. It also gives you something to discuss when you finish the books.

4. **Story Time.** Again, you don't have to share things – trade cool stories with your friends, like things that happened on summer vacation. Adults do this all the time.

# Principle 15: Loyalty

Loyalty is important. It means sticking by your friends even when annoyed with them or somebody pressurizes you. It doesn't mean you should stick with somebody who's being exceptionally mean to you or isn't loyal to you.

However, if you aren't loyal, you won't keep friends.

You must learn to stick up for your friends and stick by them. Also, learn who deserves it and who doesn't, and when loyalty means not doing what they ask. Learning loyalty will help you as you grow up.

For example, you can also be loyal to your school.

Here are some exercises to learn loyalty:

1. **Stick to Me**. Pretend you're glued to a friend. You must stay touching each other for a few minutes, walking around a room. This exercise is also physically hard.

2. **Loyalty List**. Write down all the ways you can be loyal to another person. Consider trading lists with a friend to see if you agree or where you might disagree.

3. **Trouble List**. Write down imaginary scenarios where a friend might ask you to do something. Then sort them into situations where you should be loyal, like "Let's go get ice cream," and ones where you might want to try to stop your friend, like, "Let's rob a bank." This exercise helps you remember that loyalty shouldn't be blind to your interests and theirs.

4. **Keep a Promise Diary**. Write down every commitment you make and then mark if you followed through or why you didn't. You can spot patterns and work out how to be a more loyal person by doing more of what you say you will do.

Before you move to the next section, write down four things you have learned in this chapter.

1. --------------------------------------------------------------------

2. --------------------------------------------------------------------

3. --------------------------------------------------------------------

4. --------------------------------------------------------------------

# Section 6: Finding Solutions

What do you do when you have a problem? Do you throw a tantrum, or do you look for a solution? Learning to solve problems is part of life. Learning to solve social problems means finding common ground.

Problem-solving is defined as "the process of finding solutions to difficult or complex issues." That's a lot of big words. In simpler terms, it means determining the problem and why it exists and then looking for potential solutions.

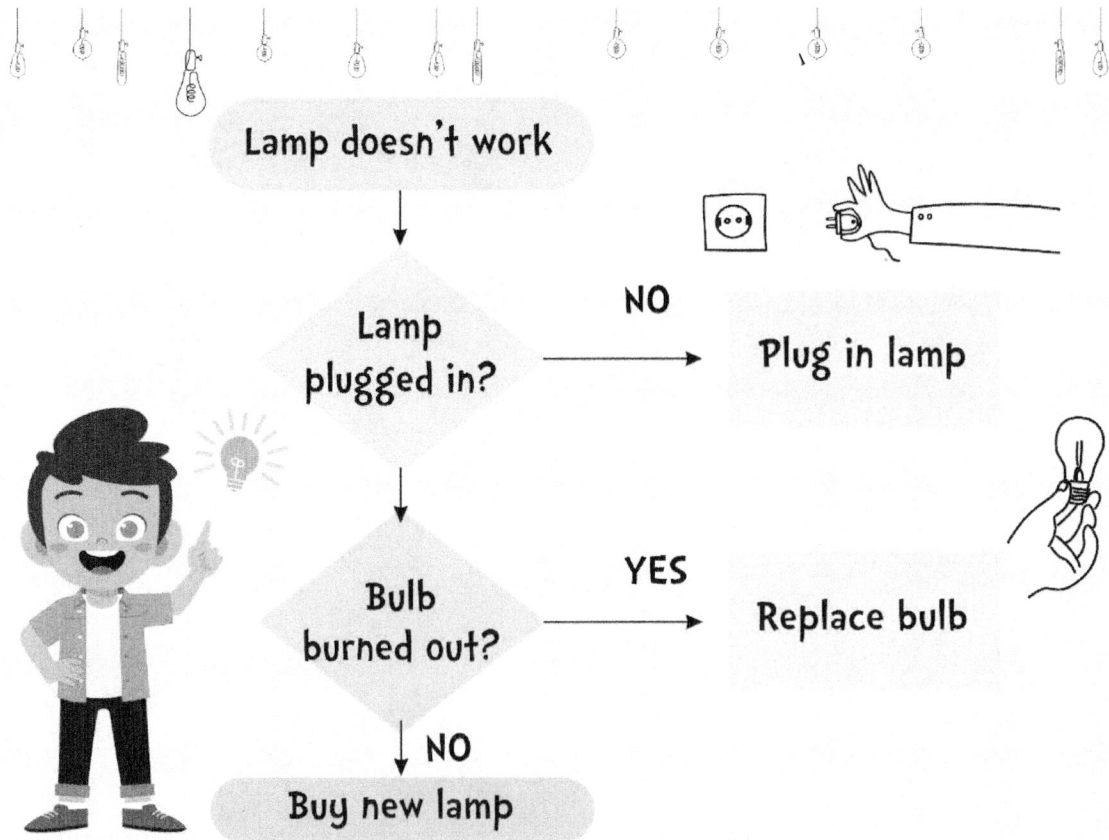

Lamp doesn't work

Lamp plugged in? → NO → Plug in lamp

Bulb burned out? → YES → Replace bulb

NO → Buy new lamp

For example, you and Marie had a fight at lunch. You both think the other was completely in the wrong. You might solve this problem by listing the ways you were each in the wrong and then finding solutions to fix your side. You might also solve it by asking somebody else to help you work things out. (This is called "mediation" and a great way to solve problems).

The three key principles for solving social problems are negotiation, compromise, and conflict resolution.

# Principle 16: Negotiation

You've probably already negotiated without knowing it. "I'll lend you my copy of Percy Jackson if..." is negotiation. You might also negotiate with your parents.

Negotiation is offering something in exchange for something else. Ideally, everyone gets something they want. Of course, sometimes, you want to let your friends share things with no strings attached. However, in life, you will need to negotiate every day.

Here are some exercises to learn to negotiate better:

1. **Play a Game Involving Trading and Negotiating Purchases**. Monopoly and Catan work well for this exercise. They're also a lot of fun.

2. **Role-Playing.** You can set up scenarios with a friend, like a pretend store, and pretend to barter with each other. Pay attention to real-life situations like negotiating which TV show to watch.

3. **List Negotiations You've Been Involved in**, for instance, negotiating more screen time to watch an educational show or negotiating who gets the corner seat at the lunch table. You will find there are a lot more than you think.

5. **The Wants Game.** Play this with a friend. Write a list of all the things you think the other person wants. Then trade your lists and tell each other how close you got.

# Principle 17: Compromise

Compromise means giving up one thing for another or something you want so a friend has what they want. Ideally, everyone compromises. However, it can be hard, and sometimes you don't want to give anything up; this is natural.

You must learn to pick your battles and acknowledge that some things are more important than others. Compromise is a key part of negotiation and conflict resolution. Remember, the aim is to make everyone as happy as possible.

Here are some compromise exercises:

1. **Compromise Examples.** Write down as many examples of compromising as you can think of. Then, think about what you would do in those situations.

2. **Block Goals.** Get some blocks and a friend. You each decide what you want to do with the blocks without telling the other. This exercise forces you to negotiate and compromise to get your desired blocks.

3. **Compromise Circle.** Create a situation. Then, draw two concentric circles with arrows out of each. Write next to the inner circle arrow, "I can't compromise," and all the things you won't budge on. Write next to the outer circle arrow, "I can compromise," and what you're willing to give.

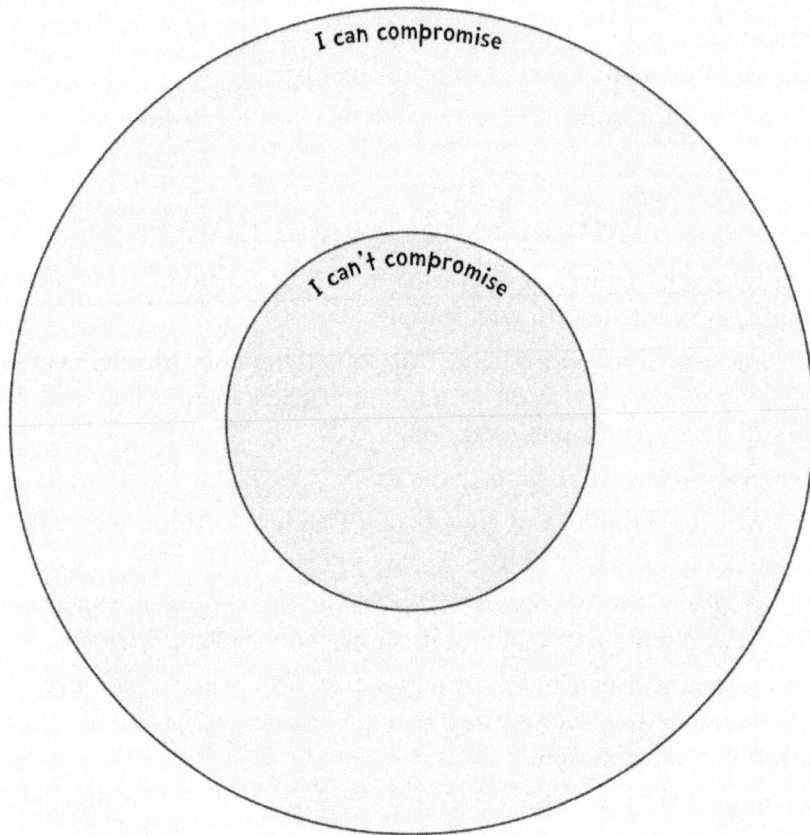

I can compromise

I can't compromise

You can then do this with a friend about an issue you struggle with, but choose a little problem, not a big one.

4.  **Pre-Conflict Exercise**. Get together with a friend, and write what you like about the other on a piece of paper, then trade them. The next time you argue, you can remind yourself of their good qualities, making compromising easier. You can do this with your parents, too.

# Principle 18: Conflict Resolution

Conflict is inevitable. Sometimes, it's caused by limited resources – for instance, there is only one copy of a book in the school library, and more than one person wants it. Sometimes, it's caused by competing needs, like one person likes the room warmer and the other colder.

Compromise and negotiation are conflict resolution elements, but ultimately, you must learn to resolve fights.

Not resolving conflict can lead to people holding long-term grudges or even throwing a punch. You've probably seen physical fights break out because people can't agree.

It's a skill you need to develop. Note you should resolve conflict, not evade it. Ignoring or evading conflict often worsens long-term or turns you into somebody everyone will take advantage of. Small problems, like your younger sister being annoying, can be ignored. But a conflict with a friend should be resolved promptly. Small conflicts can grow into big ones over time.

Here are some fun exercises to help with conflict resolution:

1. **Pushy Pairs**. Stand facing a friend. Put your arms out straight and touch your palms. Then push as hard as you can against each other (ensure you're somewhere you won't have a problem if you fall over). What does it feel like when you suddenly stop pushing? This exercise helps you visualize conflict.

2. **Conflict Resolution Journal**. Write down a conflict. Then, write down all the ways you can think of to resolve the conflict. You can include silly ones as long as you don't do them. Ask your parents or a trusted adult (if the conflict is with your parents) which is best.

3. **Big Problems Versus Little Problems**. Use the worksheet and list examples of big and little problems. Big problems generally need to involve an adult.

| Tornado! | My schedule changed | My mom's car has a flat tire | I miss my family | I'm really tired |
| My iPad fell and it broke | I missed the bus | I can't find my favorite socks | My team lost in basketball | My best friend isn't at school today |
| The teacher didn't call on me | The internet stopped working | I got injured while playing a sport | | |

| BIG PROBLEMS | MEDIUM PROBLEMS | SMALL PROBLEMS |
| --- | --- | --- |
| | | |

5. **Use the Stoplight**. When you fight with someone, close your eyes and imagine a red stoplight. Count to three before it turns yellow. This exercise helps keep you from reacting too quickly and to calm down.

# Section 7: The Confidence Code

Believing in yourself matters. You know people who are more confident and others who are less confident.

Cracking the confidence code will help you improve in school and have more friends. Real friends, not people who only want to be around you because you're "popular."

Confidence means not being afraid to be yourself but knowing your strengths. Good self-esteem affects every part of your life.

Here are some benefits:

- Better grades
- Improved mood
- Improved health
- Better relationships
- Not getting into too much trouble

Confident people love to learn and challenge themselves. When you believe in yourself and your abilities, you will want to be better in everything. You will study harder, care for yourself, and avoid trouble. Like how you protect your favorite toy, you will also protect yourself from harm because you love you! Confidence will make accepting your mistakes and failures easier so you can move on from them fast and focus on what's next. For instance, you will not be mad at yourself when you fail an exam. You know you are a good student and understand this is just one test. You will learn from your mistakes and study harder so you will do better next time.

One way to improve your self-esteem is to identify your strengths and talents.

# MY STRENGTHS

- [ ] Honest
- [ ] Good At Learning
- [ ] Good At Sharing
- [ ] Loyal
- [ ] Creative
- [ ] Kind
- [ ] Patient
- [ ] Appreciative
- [ ] Forgiving
- [ ] Empathetic
- [ ] Independent
- [ ] Thoughtful
- [ ] Trustworthy

- [ ] Grateful
- [ ] Reliable
- [ ] Determined
- [ ] Optimistic
- [ ] Insightful
- [ ] Persistent
- [ ] Cooperative
- [ ] Caring
- [ ] Hopeful
- [ ] Adventurous
- [ ] Funny
- [ ] Athletic
- [ ] A Leader

- [ ] Confident
- [ ] Non-judgmental
- [ ] Resilient
- [ ] Smart
- [ ] Curious
- [ ] A Self-starter
- [ ] Humble
- [ ] Artistic
- [ ] Helpful
- [ ] Focused
- [ ] Good At Problem Solving
- [ ] Accepting Of Others
- [ ] A Flexible Thinker

- [ ] Loving
- [ ] Capable
- [ ] Understanding
- [ ] Compassionate
- [ ] A Good Friend
- [ ] Hardworking
- [ ] Responsible
- [ ] Brave
- [ ] Talented at: _____
- [ ] Other: _____
- [ ] Other: _____
- [ ] Other: _____
- [ ] Other: _____

## My Top 3 Strengths Are:

1.
2.
3.

## Two strengths I want to develop are

_____ and _____

## Steps I can take to develop these strengths:

1.
2.
3.

1.
2.
3.

Having confidence also means you're less anxious, especially in social situations.

Three principles to help build confidence are positive self-talk, goal-setting, and assertiveness.

# Principle 19: Positive Self-Talk

People often say the worst things about themselves. Whether making fun of yourself or talking down your strengths, you talk to yourself in ways you would never talk to others.

Negative self-talk can lead to depression and low self-esteem and is a hard trap to break out of.

Developing positive self-talk habits can substantially improve your mood and confidence.

Here are some confidence exercises:

1. **Imagine You Are a Close Friend.** Say something positive the way you would say it to a friend. You are your own best friend. Talk like it.

2. **Use Affirmations.** Say something positive about yourself in the mirror every morning before or after brushing your teeth. For instance, "I'm strong" or something more specific like "I'm very good at math." Ask your parents or a friend if you're having difficulty thinking of good ones.

3. **Avoid Negative Nellies.** If someone persistently says bad things about you, they aren't your friend. Stay away from them.

4. **Evidence Check.** When you think something bad about yourself, ask if there's any evidence to prove it. If there isn't, *shut up the voice.* If there is, counter it by reminding yourself of something good about you. Perhaps you got a bad grade in chemistry but a good one in English.

# Principle 20: Goal-Setting

Grownups set goals all the time. They could be money goals, like saving for a vacation. Or they ight be hobby goals, like getting good at knitting.

Setting goals can dent your confidence if you do it wrong, but proper goal setting gives you wins to puff yourself up. Don't set goals outside your control. For example, while it's very tempting to set grades as a goal, sometimes you get a bad grade for reasons beyond your control.

When setting goals, ensure they are S.M.A.R.T. – Specific, Measurable, Attainable, Realistic, and Timely. That doesn't sound very easy, but it merely means knowing when you've achieved the goal, won't be working on it forever, and setting a goal you can reach. Break goals down into smaller parts so you can get them done faster.

Here are some goal-setting exercises:

1. **Goal Ladder.** Draw a ladder. Write your goal at the top. Then, write a step to reach that goal on each rung. You can put a sticker on the steps when you achieve them.

# MY GOAL LADDER

My Goal: _____

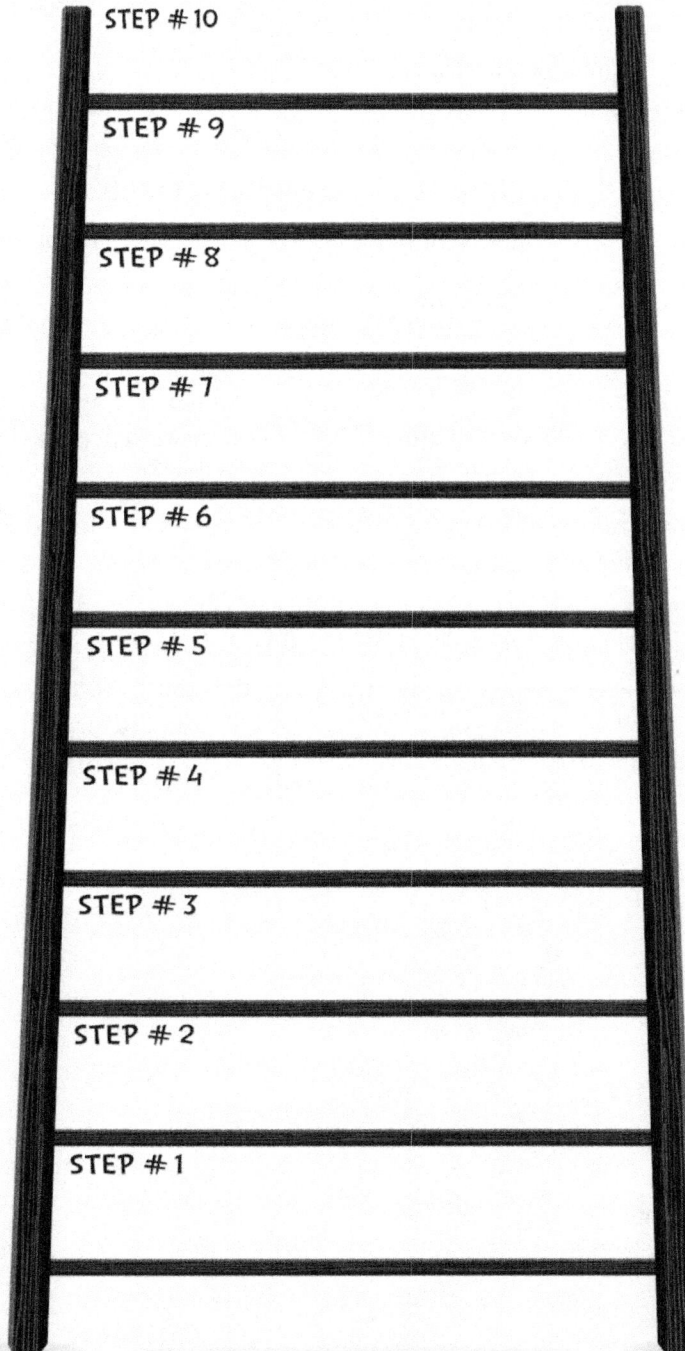

STEP #10

STEP #9

STEP #8

STEP #7

STEP #6

STEP #5

STEP #4

STEP #3

STEP #2

STEP #1

2. **Make a Bucket List.** Adults often make bucket lists of things they want to do in their lives. For children, it's better to do a shorter period, like within the next year. Share it with the adults in your life, as some things might need help to achieve.

3. **Make an Obstacles List.** Take a big goal and write down everything that might get in the way. For example, you and your parents have set a goal of hiking a nearby mountain. One obstacle might be unsuitable weather. Obstacles like the weather must be worked around by careful scheduling. Other obstacles could become mini-goals.

4. **Affirm Your Goals.** Say your goal for the day every morning so that you have it in your mind and can stay focused on it.

# Principle 21: Assertiveness

It's not wrong to be assertive. You might have been told this, especially if you're a girl. Assertiveness is good; it's aggression that's bad.

Being assertive means standing up for what you want and, in social situations, not being afraid to talk. That doesn't sound so bad, right?

It can also be scary. Most adults are afraid of public speaking because it requires being assertive. You're also probably scared to speak to the entire class. However, practicing assertiveness helps.

Here are some exercises to help you be more assertive:

1. **Practice Public Speaking.** Start small because this can be scary. Give a speech to yourself in the mirror a few times, then to your most trusted friends.

2. **Practice "I" Messages.** These are good for conflict resolution, too. "I feel that" is a great way to express your needs because it doesn't state a "fact" or put things on the other person.

3. **Passive, Aggressive, Assertive Worksheet.** Write the three columns at the top, then sort statements into each. Use words you might have said or heard or dialogue lines from a book. Show it to your parents to see what you got right.

# PASSIVE, AGGRESSIVE, AND ASSERTIVE COMMUNICATION

## Passive Communication

During passive communication, a person prioritizes the needs, wants, and feelings of others, even at their own expense. The person does not express their own needs, or does not stand up for them. This can lead to being taken advantage of, even by wellmeaning people who are unaware of the passive communicator's needs and wants.

| | |
|---|---|
| Soft spoken / quiet | Poor eye contact / looks down or away |
| Allows others to take advantage | Does not express one's own needs or wants |
| Prioritizes needs of others | Lack of confidence |

## Aggressive Communication

Through aggressive communication, a person expresses that only their own needs, wants, and feelings matter. The other person is bullied, and their needs are ignored.

| | |
|---|---|
| Easily frustrated | Use of criticism, humiliation, and domination |
| Speaks in a loud or overbearing way | Frequently interrupts or does not listen |
| Unwilling to compromise | Disrespectful toward others |

## Assertive Communication

Assertive communication emphasizes the importance of both peoples' needs. During assertive communication, a person stands up for their own needs, wants, and feelings, but also listens to and respects the needs of others. Assertive communication is defined by confidence, and a willingness to compromise.

| | |
|---|---|
| Listens without interruption | Stands up for own rights |
| Clearly states needs and wants | Confident tone / body language |
| Willing to compromise | Good eye contact |

## Examples

| | |
|---|---|
| Scenario | |
| Passive | |
| Aggressive | |
| Assertive | |

# PASSIVE, AGGRESSIVE, AND ASSERTIVE COMMUNICATION

| Scenario | Your teacher asks you to stay after school because you're behind the rest of the class. However, you have plans with your family today. |
|---|---|
| Passive | |
| Aggressive | |
| Assertive | |

| Scenario | Your sibling left a mess in your shared room, and you're too busy to clean. |
|---|---|
| Passive | |
| Aggressive | |
| Assertive | |

| Scenario | You're at a restaurant, and the server brought you the wrong dish |
|---|---|
| Passive | |
| Aggressive | |
| Assertive | |

| Scenario | A friend showed up at your house uninvited. Usually you would be happy to let them in, but this time you're busy. |
|---|---|
| Passive | |
| Aggressive | |
| Assertive | |

4. **Teach Something.** Perhaps your family has a board game none of your friends have. Get it out and teach your friends how to play. Use something you know well for confidence. Everyone has something to teach.

**Reflection Section**

a. Name five things on your bucket list.

MY BUCKET LISTS

1

2

3

4

5

b. Write five positive self-talk quotes that you used.

1

2

3

4

5

# Section 8: Respect for All

Think about your classmates. They're not all the same. You might have classmates of different races, with richer or poorer parents, or of different cultural backgrounds.

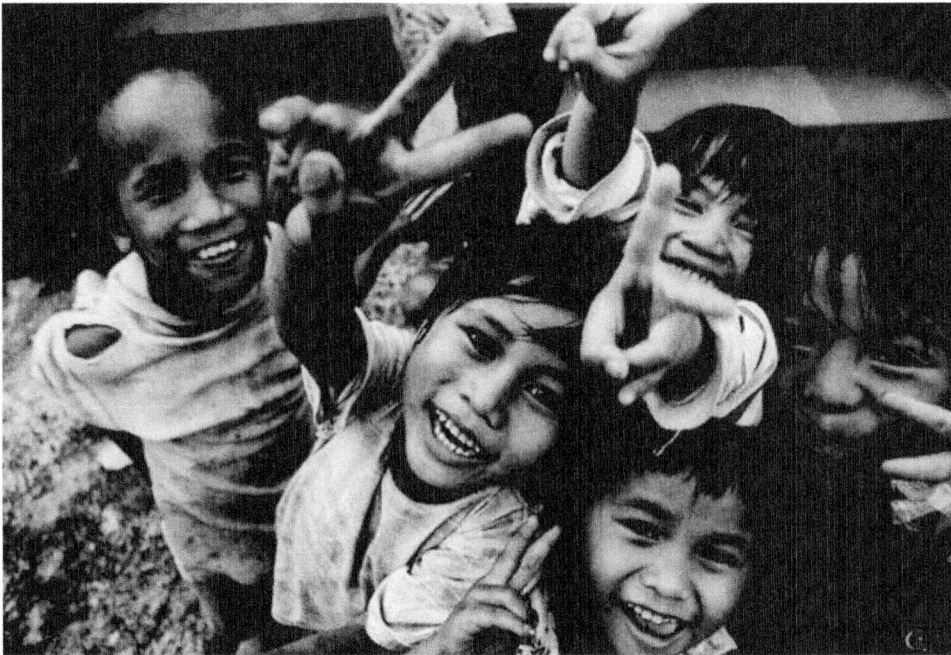

It's important to respect everyone despite your differences.

Learning to respect everyone despite their differences is a challenge. Many adults never manage it, so starting now will help you be a better person.

You must learn to avoid stereotypes and assumptions, including ones you might hear from adults. Question any statement that starts with "All" or "Those people." No group of people is "all" anything.

Treat everyone with kindness. Listen when they talk about themselves. Different cultures should be appreciated and valued.

The three principles are accepting differences, cultural sensitivity, and respect for others' beliefs.

# Principle 22: Accepting Differences

"That boy's weird." You might have heard this before. Other children will often decide somebody is weird because they act differently. It might be that they are autistic. Or they might be immigrants from another country still working on their English.

Learning to accept differences doesn't mean ignoring or tolerating them but embracing them.

It can help to see what you have in common. The child who just moved from Germany might have a strong accent and an annoying younger sibling. You can bond over common things while accepting those that are different.

Here are some fun things you can do:

1.  **Research Another Culture**. If you are researching a classmate's culture, ask them polite questions about it. Share stories about your family's traditions in return.

2.  **Read a Book with a Main Character Very Different from You**. Ask your school librarian for advice.

3.  **Create a Difference Collage**. Get old magazines, cut out pictures of different people, and put them on a poster board. Hang it where you can be reminded of respecting cultural differences. Ask for help if needed.

4.  **Get Together with Friends and Make a Diversity Quilt**. Each person draws something representing their culture on the quilt.

# Principle 23: Cultural Sensitivity

More big words. It means you must understand people have different cultures and not "rank" them. Many people put their culture on top.

People also do "exoticizing," looking at somebody else's culture and seeing it as neat or cool. You shouldn't dress up in somebody else's culture for Halloween; they might be offended.

Cultural sensitivity starts by understanding that everyone has a culture. Your family has its own mini-culture – think of things you do differently from your friends.

Some exercises to learn cultural sensitivity:

1. **Listen to Songs in Other Languages**. YouTube has many songs in almost every language, or have your parents find them for you. The music is understandable, but the words are not. Are these songs better or worse than those you listen to? Or are they just different?

2. **Read Folk Tales from Other Cultures**. For example, ask your parents to find you different versions of Cinderella. Did you know there's a Chinese Cinderella and an Indian one?

3. **Practice Names**. It can be hard to pronounce unfamiliar names. Rude people assign nicknames to overcome learning to pronounce them properly. Start with your classmates' names or work on the names of famous people – your favorite foreign actor, sports idol, or boy band.

4. **Learn Phrases in Other Languages**. You could learn to say thank you in a whole bunch of languages, reminding you that everyone communicates.

# Principle 24: Respect for Others' Beliefs

Does your family go to church? Or synagogue? Other people have different beliefs, not only about God(s). They might also have different ideas about family life, how the universe is put together, or what is okay to eat and what shouldn't be eaten.

Respecting others' beliefs is important as long as they don't harm you. You don't necessarily have to respect the person who keeps trying to convert you because they aren't respecting you, and it has to go both ways.

Perhaps you have a friend who's a vegetarian. You should not keep trying to get them to eat fried chicken.

Some exercises to encourage respect for other beliefs:

1. **Research Somebody Else's Religion**. Consider going to their place of worship and (politely) looking around. A Hindu temple looks very different from a Methodist church.

2. **List Your Values**. Knowing your values helps you respect other people's values. Write down whether you believe in God, how you feel about eating animals, etc. Talk to your parents about this, too. Your values will overlap with theirs but also might not.

3. **Trade Values**. With a close friend, each should write down what they think the other values. This exercise helps you deal with assumptions, understand each other better, and see things about yourself.

4. **Draw a Religion Tree**. On the trunk, put things most religions have in common. On the branches put things which are different. You notice basics like "Help people in need" are

common, even to other beliefs like atheism. Branches are typically things like "Celebrates Hanukkah" or "Wears henna when getting married."

## RELIGION TREE

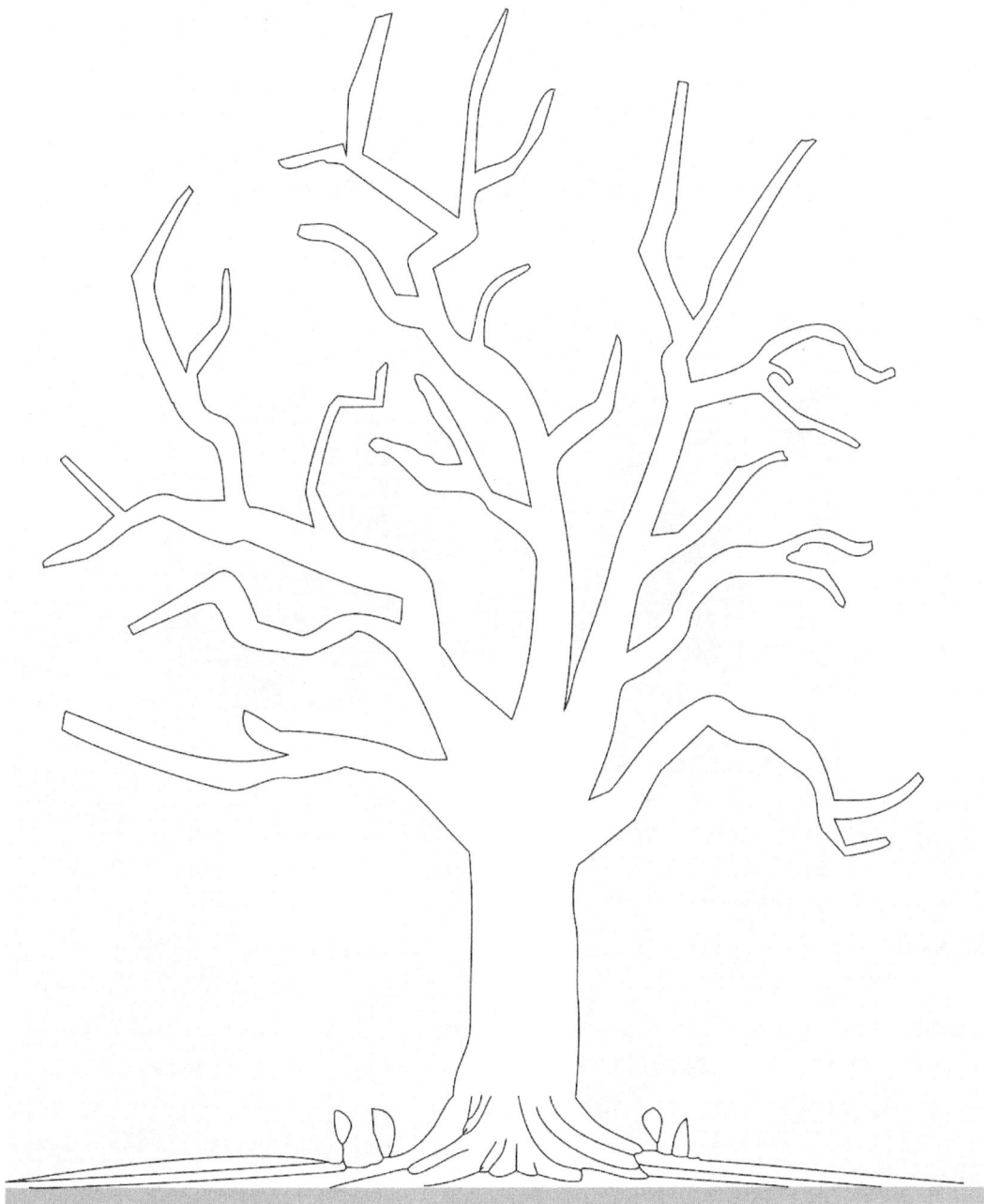

# Section 9: Dealing with Bullying

Have you been bullied? Do you know any bullies? Bullying is common, and a lot of children do it or fall victim to it.

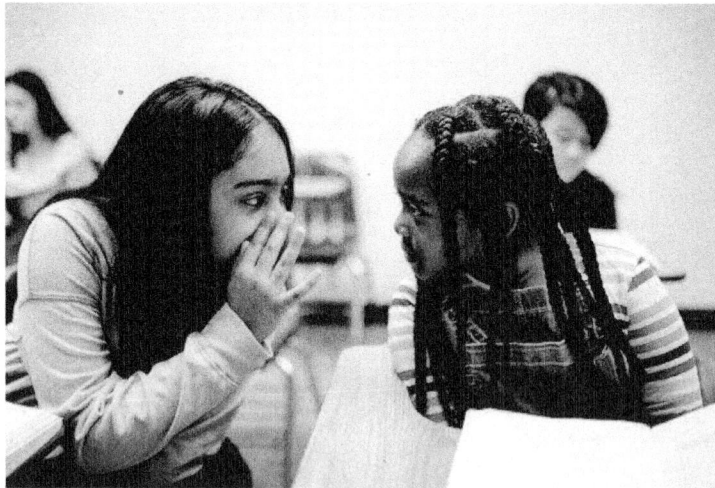

Bullying has many different forms.

Some children just aren't very nice. A common mistake is to think it's only bullying if it is hitting or shoving. However, bullying can take different forms:

- **Physical.** Hitting, shoving, hair pulling, etc. Physical bullying can escalate into fights, causing serious damage, including injuries and damage to property, like breaking somebody's glasses.

- **Verbal.** Insulting people, saying nasty things to their faces, including using bad words about race, gender, or physical appearance. Verbal bullying impacts self-esteem.

- **Social.** When the bully tries to damage your relationships with others. For example, threatening somebody if they hang out with you. It results in your being isolated, causing social anxiety if successful.

- **Cyberbullying.** Internet bullying can fall under verbal or social but deserves its own category because it's often harder to deal with.

Social bullying can be tough to recognize, as the person being bullied often does not see it happen. It can sometimes be hard to notice you're doing it yourself.

The three principles for dealing with bullying are recognizing, reporting, and refusing. These steps create a safe place where bullying isn't tolerated.

# Principle 25: Recognize

Sometimes, it's very easy to recognize bullying. A bigger child forcing a smaller one to give them a candy bar is easy to notice.

However, sometimes, it's a lot harder.

Here are some exercises to help:

1. **Bully or Buddy.** The worksheet has you mark each statement as bullying or being nice (buddy).

## BUDDY OR BULLY?

Read each statement. If it describes a buddy, color in the happy face.
If it describes a bully, color in the mean face.

Cares about how other people feel.

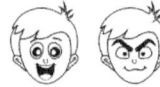

Laughs when other people mess up.

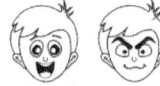

Takes turns and shares.

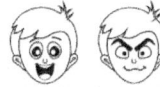

Plays with everyone.

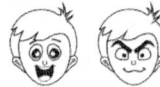

Is kind and respectful.

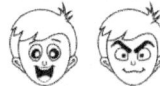

Tries to make others look dumb or not cool.

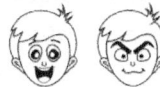

Uses polite or nice words.

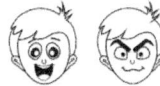

Pushes, hits or punches other people.

Calls people mean names.

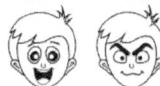

Helps other people.

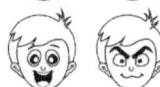

2. **Learn the Signs That Your Friends Might Be Being Bullied.** Not only the signs that somebody hit them but also if you see somebody hiding behind the teacher, sitting alone, or avoiding activities, they might be bullied.

3. **Bullying Thermometer.** Some bullying is worse than others. Some are worse to some people than others. Some children might handle being shoved better than being called names. Write down different bullying types, then arrange them from cool (not too bad) to hot (terrible). Have a friend do it, too, and compare – for example, name-calling, spreading rumors, and punching.

4. **Brainstorm Why You Think Bullies Do It.** Do they want to feel more powerful? Be accepted? Avoid being bullied themselves? Bullies have reasons.

# Principle 26: Report

Bullying keeps happening when adults never find out about it. You might be afraid to report the bully in case they retaliate (try to get you back!). Or you might be embarrassed because the bullying seems so stupid.

You might also think adults won't do anything.

Your school should have an anti-bullying policy. Read it or have your parents explain it to you. If all else fails, talk to your parents. They can help you. You don't have only to report bullying happening to you. You should report bullying that you know is happening to others. For example, if somebody is spreading nasty rumors about Christine, you should report it.

However, the hardest part is not wanting to report it. These exercises to practice reporting will help you:

1. **Role-Play.** Create an imaginary bullying scenario with a trusted friend, then tell your friend about it. It allows you to practice reporting and makes it easier to tell an adult.

2. **"It's Not My Fault."** The goal of the bully is to make you feel ashamed and helpless. It's a lot easier to report bullying if you don't feel this way. Repeat "It's not my fault" to yourself until you believe it, and it will be much easier to report. You did nothing wrong. The bully did.

3. **Write Down the Steps to Report Bullying at Your School.** Writing something down makes it easier to remember. For example, make a list of talking to a teacher, your parents, etc.

4. **Use Affirmations.** Say three good things about yourself every morning. Many children don't report bullying because they convince themselves they deserve it.

# Principle 27: Refuse

Refusing is sticking up to the bully, but that's not always safe. For example, you should try not to fight back. One favorite trick of bullies is to provoke you into throwing the first punch and then report you for fighting. Only push back physically if you're attacked and need to defend yourself.

Refusing means two things:

- Don't let the bully get to you if you can avoid it. Staying calm and not reacting emotionally can sometimes get them to change targets.

- Don't participate. Don't be part of the problem.

For example, if somebody's trying to get you to shun another person who hasn't done anything to you, don't go along with it. If you have to choose, don't choose the bully, no matter how much it might hurt. Sometimes, the bully is your friend, or you think they are.

Here are some exercises and tips for refusing bullies:

1. **Use the Block Button.** If you're being bullied on Facebook or another social app, block them. Do this after saving everything they say to you. Encourage your friends to do the same.

2. **Learn "Bully Bans."** Talk this one over with your parents. These are short statements you memorize and can then pull out when you see somebody being bullied. They might include "You're over the line," "Knock it off," or "Whatever." Practice them.

3. **Change the Subject.** Practice this one with your friends. If somebody's being verbally bullied, start a different conversation. Ask about the score of the last football game, the weather, or something that happened in class.

4. **Do a Kind Thing.** Do something nice for the person being bullied. Wave at them. Offer to sit next to them. You can help them feel better and stand up for themselves.

# Section 10: Bringing It All Together

Everything in this book works together. Think of it as a whole, not 27 different parts.

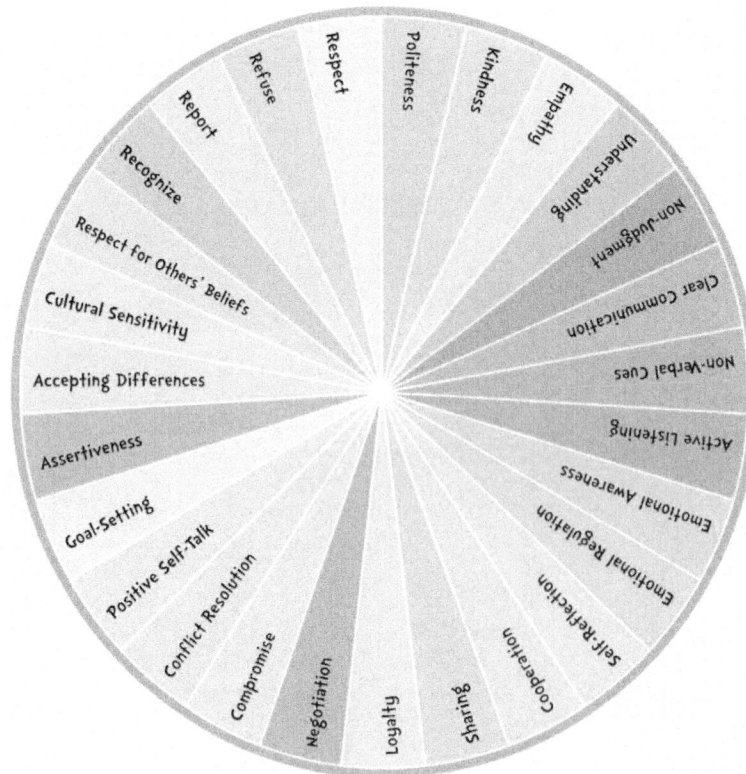

So, how do they connect? Look at the diagram above; you'll see lines connecting them. For example, self-reflection helps you refuse bullies. Positive self-talk helps you not judge others.

So, here are a few exercises to bring it all together:

1. **Emotion Charades.** Write emotions down, pick one, and then act it out for your friends. This combines emotional awareness and nonverbal communication.

2. **Brainstorm What Makes a Good Friend**. Make a list with your friends. This helps you work on loyalty, positive self-talk, and recognizing bullying.

3. **Play the Sorry Game**. Create a scenario, then sort possible apologies into real or fake. This helps you work on negotiation, clear communication, and conflict resolution.

4. **Play the Teasing Game**. You want to do this with somebody you truly trust. One of you teases the other, and the other must not react or must practice walking away. This helps you both recognize and refuse bullying and what not to say.

Remember, you're practicing social skills whenever you talk to anyone, at school or at home. Sometimes, it makes it easy to interact with others if you think about how much you're learning.

**Exercise**

Now that you have finished the book, write down all the lessons you have learned.

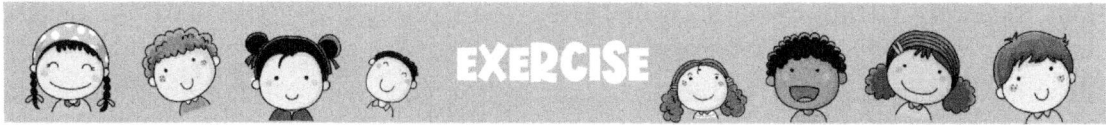

EXERCISE

--------------------------------------------------

--------------------------------------------------

--------------------------------------------------

--------------------------------------------------

--------------------------------------------------

--------------------------------------------------

--------------------------------------------------

--------------------------------------------------

--------------------------------------------------

--------------------------------------------------

--------------------------------------------------

--------------------------------------------------

--------------------------------------------------

--------------------------------------------------

--------------------------------------------------

--------------------------------------------------

--------------------------------------------------

--------------------------------------------------

# Thank You Message

Learning better social skills is hard. Thank you for working on it.

Did you enjoy reading the book? Although there are fun and cool activities, there are also interesting lessons that you shouldn't forget. The book gave you all the information you need to understand the world of social interactions. For example, if you want to know if someone is angry, actively listen to them and notice their non-verbal cues. You can also train yourself to be more empathetic to feel people's pain. Through empathy, you can build healthy and strong relationships. The book also covered emotional intelligence and showed you how to understand and regulate your emotions.

The main rule in socializing is connecting with people. The book explains certain qualities like sharing, cooperation, and loyalty so you can better communicate and connect with others.

You know how your parents always tell you: for every problem, there is a solution. However, sometimes you can't find it. The book showed you how to resolve conflict, compromise, and negotiate to solve problems.

If you want to be happy and make friends, you should always respect others and make them feel loved. In this book, you learned how to embrace other people's differences and treat them with kindness. All the lessons in this book will help you now and later in your life. So use it as a guide and keep coming back to it whenever you are struggling and need help.

Thank you for buying this book. Hopefully, you will take away from it tools to help you through your life. Adults have all these problems, too, except they are often bigger. This book will help you journey down the right path.

But you have to do the rest yourself: listening to others, setting goals, and, above all, being kind.

If you think about being kind first, the rest will often follow. Thank you for being kind.

# Check out another book in the series

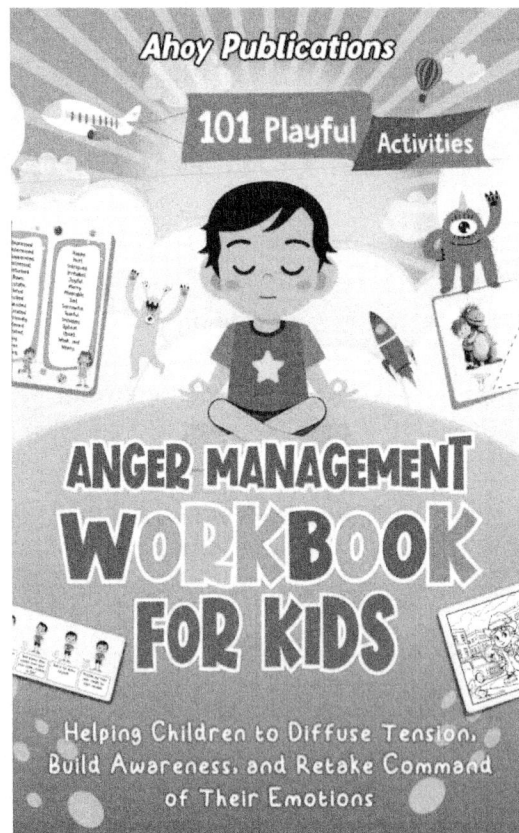

# References

And, C. (n.d.). Cultural Sensitivity. Nyc.gov. https://www.nyc.gov/assets/ochia/downloads/pdf/cultural_sensitivity_wkshp.pdf

Fell, A. (2022, April 15). Research review shows self-esteem has long-term benefits. UC Davis. https://www.ucdavis.edu/curiosity/news/research-review-shows-self-esteem-has-long-term-benefits

Guerra-Bustamante, J., León-del-Barco, B., Yuste-Tosina, R., López-Ramos, V. M., & Mendo-Lázaro, S. (2019). Emotional intelligence and psychological well-being in adolescents. International Journal of Environmental Research and Public Health, 16(10), 1720. https://doi.org/10.3390/ijerph16101720

Lebow, H. I. (2016, May 17). Emotional intelligence (EQ): Components and tips. Psych Central. https://psychcentral.com/lib/what-is-emotional-intelligence-eq

Volpe, A. (2022, July 6). How to be a little less judgmental. Vox. https://www.vox.com/even-better/23188518/be-less-judgmental-tips

What is active listening? (n.d.). United States Institute of Peace. https://www.usip.org/public-education-new/what-active-listening

Bryant, Colleen Doyle. "What Is Empathy?" *Talking with Trees Books*, https://talkingtreebooks.com/teaching-resources-catalog/definitions/what-is-empathy.html#:~:text=Empathy%20is%20being%20able%20to%20know%20how%20someone%20else%20is,see%20things%20from%20their%20view.

"Why Building Confidence Can Benefit Learners and Help Them to Achieve." *NCFE*, www.ncfe.org.uk/all-articles/confidence-benefits-learners/.

Printed in Dunstable, United Kingdom